D0101972

Making a Difference with Nursing Research

Rae Langford, EdD, MS, BS
Professor
Texas Woman's University
College of Nursing

Anne Young, EdD, MS, BS
Professor
Texas Woman's University
College of Nursing

PEARSON

Boston   Columbus   Indianapolis   New York   San Francisco   Upper Saddle River
Amsterdam   Cape Town   Dubai   London   Madrid   Milan   Munich   Paris   Montréal   Toronto
Delhi   Mexico City   São Pa   Singapore   Taipei   Tokyo

HANLEY LIBRARY

B01452K2036

Editor in Chief: Julie Alexander
Acquisitions Editor: Pamela Fuller
Editorial Project Manager: Patrick Walsh
Editorial Assistant: Cynthia Gates
Director of Marketing: David Gesell
Senior Marketing Manager: Phoenix Harvey
Marketing Manager: Debi Doyle
Development Editor: Karla Paschkis
Production Project Manager: Debbie Ryan
Art Director: Jayne Conte

Cover Designer: Bruce Kenselaar
Art Director Interior: Maria Guglielmo-Walsh
Interior Designer: Dina Curro
Cover Art: Fotolia
Lead Media Project Manager: Rachel Collett
Full-Service Project Management: Chitra Ganesan
Composition: PreMediaGlobal
Printer/Binder: R.R. Donnelley/Crawfordsville
Cover Printer: Lehigh-Phoenix Color/Hagerstown
Text Font: Times LT Std Roman 10/12

Microsoft® and Windows® are registered trademarks of the Microsoft Corporation in the U.S.A. and other countries. Screen shots and icons reprinted with permission from the Microsoft Corporation. This book is not sponsored or endorsed by or affiliated with the Microsoft Corporation.

Copyright © 2013 by Pearson Education, Inc. All rights reserved. Manufactured in the United States of America. This publication is protected by Copyright, and permission should be obtained from the publisher prior to any prohibited reproduction, storage in a retrieval system, or transmission in any form or by any means, electronic, mechanical, photocopying, recording, or likewise. To obtain permission(s) to use material from this work, please submit a written request to Pearson Education, Inc., Permissions Department, One Lake Street, Upper Saddle River, New Jersey 07458, or you may fax your request to 201-236-3290.

Many of the designations by manufacturers and sellers to distinguish their products are claimed as trademarks. Where those designations appear in this book, and the publisher was aware of a trademark claim, the designations have been printed in initial caps or all caps.

Catalogue in Publication data available from the Library of Congress.

PEARSON

Education

This book is not for sale or distribution in the U.S.A. or Canada

2000317

10 9 8 7 6 5 4 3 2 1

Edge Hill University
Learning Services

Barcode 265658

PEARSON

ISBN 10: 0-13-234399-1
ISBN 13: 978-0-13-234399-2

About the Authors

Rae Langford   I am a professor at Texas Woman's University College of Nursing—Houston Center. I have taught research and statistics to undergraduate students, graduate students, and practitioners in nursing for more than 35 years. My goal as I work with various courses at various levels is to make research more readily applicable in nursing practice by making materials clear, readily understood, and easily accessible, and by making learning experiences relevant and fun. I firmly believe that students learn when given the right tools and practical opportunities to learn how to learn.

Anne Young   I am a professor at Texas Woman's University College of Nursing—Houston Center and teach research and nursing education courses. As a nurse educator for over 30 years, I actively supervise students completing doctoral dissertation research. My nursing research focuses primarily on educational testing and end of life issues. I have always wanted to make a difference for patients and families who require nursing care. It is particularly gratifying to facilitate students as they learn how to conduct and use nursing research. It is my goal to help nurses and nursing students at all levels make nursing research a critical part of their practice.

We hope that you, the student, find these materials useful and relevant as you embark on your journey to learn the research process and to apply research findings to enhance the care that you offer to your patients.

This book is dedicated to our mother,
Mae Wynelle Shackelford Langford—
A nurse who shared her love
of nursing with her daughters.

Reviewers

Thank You

Our heartfelt thanks go out to our colleagues from schools of nursing across the country who have given their time generously to help us create this exciting new edition of our book. We have reaped the benefit of your collective experience as nurses and teachers, and we have made many improvements due to your efforts. Among those who gave us their encouragement and comments are:

Janet G. Alexander, EdD, MSN, RN
Professor, Samford University
Birmingham, AL

Marilyn E. Asselin, PhD, RN-BC
Assistant Professor, University
of Massachusetts Dartmouth
North Dartmouth, MA

Dot Baker, RN, MS(N), CNS-BC, EdD
Professor, Wilmington University
Georgetown, DE

Martha Baker, PhD, RN, CNE, ACNS-BC
Professor, Southwest Baptist University
Springfield, MO

Sharon E. Beck, BSN, RN Ed.M, MSN, PhD
Adjunct Professor, Thomas Edison State
College, Drexel University,
Brandman University, CA

Angeline Bushy, PhD, RN, FAAN
Professor, University of Central Florida
Daytona Beach, FL

Lynn Clark Callister, RN, PhD, FAAN
Professor, Brigham Young University
Provo, UT

Lynda Cessario, RN, PhD
Assistant Professor, Daemen College
Amherst, NY

Carolyn Hoffman, PhD, RN, CPNP
Assistant Professor,
University of Louisville
Louisville, KY

Zena Hyman, RN, ANP-BC, MS
Adjunct Professor, Daemen College
Amherst, NY

Susan Miovech, PhD, RNC
Associate Professor,
Holy Family University
Philadelphia, PA

Patricia A. Ottani
Associate Professor, Saint Anselm College
Manchester, NH

Mary Carol G. Pomatto, EdD, ARNP-CNS
Professor/Department Chair,
Pittsburg State University
Pittsburg, KS

Susan P. Porterfield, PhD FNP-C
Assistant Professor,
Florida State University
Tallahassee, FL

Ellen Rich, PhD, RN, FNP
Associate Professor, Molloy College
Rockville Centre, NY

Sheryl Samuelson, PhD, RN
Associate Professor, Milkin University
Decatur, IL

Rose Schecter, PhD, RN
Professor, Molloy College
Rockville Centre, NY

Theresa Skybo, PhD, RN, CPNP
Assistant Professor, Ohio State University
Columbus, OH

Molly J. Walker, PhD, RN, CNS, CNE
Associate Professor,
Angelo State University
San Angelo, TX

Elaine Yellen, PhD, RN
Associate Professor, Texas A&M University
College Station, TX

Preface

You may be asking yourselves *Why is RESEARCH a required course? What does RESEARCH have to do with being a nurse?* The American Nurses Association considers research so important to nursing that it expects all registered nurses to receive educational preparation about how to read and understand the research literature and to learn how it can be applied to the practice of nursing.

This textbook and companion web site are designed to enhance your skills so that you can read, understand, and apply research findings in your clinical practice. The book is divided into three sections. Part 1 is comprised of Chapters 1 through 3. This section introduces you to the concept of nursing research and where nursing as a profession has been and where it is going in the use and production of research. You will learn about databases and search strategies and useful research resources so that you can successfully find research evidence. Finally, you examine the definition of research and are introduced to the research process.

Chapters 4 through 7 comprise Part 2. Part 2 is designed to give you the vocabulary and background necessary to read and understand research studies. You will be introduced to two broad research traditions known as qualitative and quantitative research and learn how they differ from one another. Chapters 5 and 6 will then give you a close-up and personal view of the quantitative research process and will investigate different types of quantitative research. Chapter 7 will give you a more in-depth look at types of qualitative research and the qualitative research process.

Part 3 is comprised of Chapters 8, 9, and 10. This section is designed to help you acquire the necessary skills to apply what you have learned in the first two sections. Here you will get step by step guidance in how to effectively read and understand actual research articles. You will be introduced to an evidence-based practice model that will help you to identify relevant clinical problems and collect and evaluate research evidence on those problems, and then guide you in applying what you have found in the clinical area. There is an entire chapter that walks you through the evidence-based practice process using a sample clinical problem.

Chapter Features

You will find helpful features in each chapter. All chapters provide a quick overview right up front including an outline, chapter objectives, key vocabulary terms, and a chapter abstract. This allows you to see what the chapter is all about at a glance. You will also find several innovations to make the whole research process easier to understand. Boxed materials provide examples from real research articles to illustrate the various research steps and *Consider This* boxes pose questions for you to think about as you read. *Research in the News* uses stories straight from a variety of newspapers that show how healthcare research is reported in our everyday lives. Bulleted summaries give you a quick review of key points and are tied to the chapter objectives. There are two sets of activities that you may use to help you further explore the materials that you have just read about. One set is listed at the end of each chapter and is labeled *Student Activities*. There are also more activities on the companion web site for this book. So have a little fun with your learning.

You may find that you not only learn how to effectively use research in your nursing practice, but that you also gain greater abilities to read and think critically, to analyze situations, and to better use and manage available resources. We invite you now to begin your journey into the world of nursing research.

Acknowledgements

We thank our editors at Pearson, Pamela Fuller and Karla Paschkis, for their assistance and perseverance with the process of producing this book.

Contents

What's It All About?

. . . a professional expectation, a role, a connection to nursing's past and future, an emerging process

We live in an age where information flourishes. We have unprecedented access to information on almost any subject. You just enter a phrase in the computer search line and a million of hits appear instantly on the screen. Such power, but it can all be very overwhelming at times. In fact such overload can confuse and weigh us down and may make us fail to use this wealth of information to our best advantage. We need a way to make this information explosion work for us. How? We need to hone the necessary skills to define what information we need and to determine how to find and use that information. This section is designed to help you do that. It introduces you to research and the research process and teaches you about useful resources for this content and how to best access and use those resources.

Research in Nursing—An Overview

CHAPTER OUTLINE

CHAPTER OBJECTIVES

1. Discuss the mechanisms used to acquire knowledge.
2. Define the basic characteristics of research and nursing research.
3. Trace important historical events in nursing research.
4. Link educational level to nursing roles in research.
5. Describe the role of evidence-based practice in clinical nursing.
6. Describe priorities for nursing research.
7. Discuss facilitators and barriers to conducting and using nursing research.

KEY TERMS

Authority (**p. 4**)

Consumer of research
(**p. 15**)

Deductive reasoning (**p. 4**)

Evidence-based practice
(**p. 16**)

Inductive reasoning (**p. 4**)

Intuition (**p. 4**)

Multidisciplinary research
(**p. 16**)

Nurse scientist (**p. 15**)

Nursing research (**p. 5**)

Personal experience (**p. 4**)

Research (**p. 5**)

Traditional practice (**p. 4**)

Translational research
(**p. 16**)

Trial and error (**p. 4**)

ABSTRACT

When new health discoveries and technologies emerge, nursing care practices change in response. Nurses want to offer their patients the very best care available. To do that, they must identify the best sources of information about nursing care and use that information to develop a solid, scientific basis for care delivery. Although there are many sources of information, research is the only one that utilizes a systematic process of discovery and testing.

Nursing has a rich history of discovery that has the potential to guide practice. Regardless of the level of education, all nurses have a place in the world of nursing research, whether it is to generate new knowledge or apply research findings to practice. Evidence-based practice is a practical method for applying research findings to nursing practice. While some barriers exist, there is a bright future for engaging in nursing research and applying the findings—activities that will benefit patient care.

What Is Research?

Imagine a world where things are constantly changing. People want to figure out how things work. They want to explain what is happening around them. In ancient times, people saw the sun come up and go down, they saw the moon and stars in the night sky, they felt the storms that periodically arose and passed through. How did they explain these phenomena? Throughout the ages people have always searched for answers. In ancient times, wise people or "authorities" crafted answers and passed them down to others. Traditions, based on the best understanding available, were created for how to do things. Sometimes people figured things out by using their common sense and their past experiences. Other times the process of trial and error helped people try things again and again until they worked. Over time, more systematic discovery methods developed that used logic and investigation. From those humble beginnings, science evolved into the enterprise that we have today. This chapter explains what research is and why it matters. It explores the history of nursing research, nursing research roles, the emergence of evidence-based practice (EBP), and most importantly, the future of research.

How Do We Know What Is Real?

Nursing has also used many sources of knowledge to guide practice. Nurses have used **traditional practices** as a part of nursing care: these are practices handed down from one group of nurses to the next. Oftentimes, traditional practices are included as part of the information taught in nursing programs. Using tradition means not having to reinvent the wheel for every clinical problem encountered. The problem with this approach is that a practice can be traditional without having been verified as effective. For instance, it used to be traditional to keep surgery patients in bed for several days following their procedures. As the negative effects of immobility were discovered, a more active program of science-based early activity was implemented.

Authority has also served as a source of knowledge for nursing practices. In school, students depend on teachers to share information about clinical practices. Textbooks and journals are considered authoritative sources. In clinical settings, students and new nurses may ask more experienced nurses or other health care providers how a particular clinical problem should be managed and trust in their experience and judgment. While consultation with authorities facilitates practice, a downside is that the information provided by authorities may not have been systematically tested.

Personal experience is the knowledge nurses gain through practice that often guides clinical decisions. Nurses may think back to the last time they encountered a similar clinical problem and then make a decision about managing a comparable clinical problem based on that past experience. Acquiring experience is critical to nursing decisions and helps individuals to gain expertise as nurses, but it has limiting features as well. Experiences may be subjective, based on personal values and perceptions. It may be difficult to pass on information based on personal experiences to others who have not had a similar experience. Also, individuals have a limited number of experiences and may consequently encounter new situations with which they are not familiar. **Intuition** regarding clinical situations is closely related to and may draw on personal experiences. Here, a person follows a hunch about a particular situation to guide their actions. Benner (1984) indicates that expert nurses intuitively grasp situations based on their deep understanding of past similar situations.

Trial and error allows solving problems simply by thinking of alternatives and trying them out until one works. While this can be a practical means of problem solving in some instances, it is inefficient and unsystematic. Even worse, solutions found through trial and error can be shared with only a limited number of people since this information is usually transmitted person to person rather than through literature or other broad-based communication sources.

Reasoning represents another way to figure things out. Reasoning requires the use of analytical abilities to think about how to solve a problem. **Inductive reasoning** moves from specific information to general principles while **deductive reasoning** moves from general principles to specific situations. For example, using inductive reasoning, a nurse might note that pain control is of critical concern to the patients he/she cares for when they return from surgical procedures. Based on these specific observations, the nurse concludes that postoperative pain from incisions and tissue manipulation is a common occurrence that must be managed for all surgical patients. Using deductive reasoning, a nurse might work from the general premise that surgical procedures cause trauma to tissue that in turn generates pain. Therefore, the nurse concludes that pain management will be an important postoperative measure for each surgical patient. Both inductive and deductive reasoning provide means of understanding and responding to clinical situations. Each type of reasoning plays a role in research. Yet reasoning also has shortcomings. For one thing, individuals may not have sufficient accurate information to correctly deduce what appropriate actions might be. For another, individuals may not have sufficient experience with individual cases to correctly draw a larger conclusion.

All of these strategies are useful in clinical situations in that they allow nurses to deal with clinical problems on a day-to-day basis. Yet they all share a serious shortcoming: they are not supported by systematic study to ensure that the practices promote the desired effect.

Systematic Discovery—The Process of Research

Consider This . . .

When you hear the word research, what pops into your head? Describe what the word means to you.

Research means discovery, especially systematic discovery. So, how does this discovery differ from other forms of discovery discussed earlier? Exactly what is research, and more specifically, what is nursing research? Research has many definitions, most of which have overlapping components. Langford (2001) defines **research** as a "systematic process using both inductive and deductive reasoning to confirm and refine existing knowledge and to build new knowledge" (p. 72). Let's explore each component of this definition in more detail. *Systematic* implies that research that is carried out in a precise and organized manner. Following guidelines systematically increases the objectivity and accuracy of data collection. Research is a *process*, a planned series of steps used for gathering and analyzing information. Chapter 3 discusses the research process in more detail. When nurses use *inductive reasoning* in research, they may raise issues regarding specific clinical problems and seek to design studies that test assumptions about what they know from clinical practice in order to apply them more broadly. Using *deductive reasoning* allows nurses to test practice theories by applying them to a specific clinical problem. *Confirm* means verifying a belief or theory through systematic investigation. *Refine* indicates that research can assist, enhance, or improve the knowledge base by further expanding the current understanding of a phenomenon. The ultimate outcome of research is an expanded knowledge base. It strives for objectivity and freedom from bias. Research engages in a checks-and-balances system in which others scrutinize studies and outcomes to ensure that bias was minimized to the greatest extent possible.

Research is a generic term that applies to systematic discovery in many disciplines. Nursing research is any research that addresses the concerns of nursing. Thus, **nursing research** is a systematic process that helps nurses discover answers and resolve problems that are important to clinical practice, administration, or education.

Knowledge Nurses Can Use

Why is research considered so important to the world of nursing? The bottom line is that research increases nursing's science-based knowledge, which in turn improves the quality of care that patients and their families receive. Nursing research provides a mechanism for systematically and objectively analyzing practices that matter to nursing. Please keep in mind that nursing research focuses on different concerns than medical research. Although nursing and medicine work together and harmonize with one another, the central focus of what nursing does remains unique. Nursing focuses its research on human beings as individuals, as members of social groups, and as families (Donaldson 2000). Oftentimes, nursing concerns are the ones with the most impact on the day-to-day, moment-to-moment management of events happening in patients' lives. The scope of nursing research ranges from health promotion and disease prevention to care during illness or at the end of life. The substance of nursing research has grown. For example, nursing research has made incredible progress in raising consciousness about pain management, to the extent that pain assessment has become the fifth vital sign. Nurses have also investigated restraint use and incontinence control, producing findings that have significantly altered practice. For example, by building on the earlier work of nurse researchers who investigated urinary incontinence, using practical measuring devices for pelvic muscle function, and investigating the effectiveness of pelvic muscle exercises to prevent incontinence, Lajiness, Wolfert, Hall, Sampselle, and Diokno (2007) successfully demonstrated that nurse-taught pelvic muscle floor training and bladder training programs helped over 90% of their participants improve or resolve their urinary incontinence. Another example of research-driven practice modifications is restraint use. In response to findings by Strumpf and Evans (1988), many institutions began changing their policies regarding restraint use. Winston, Morelli, Bramble, Friday, and Sanders (1999) described reductions in restraint use through a nurse-driven protocol of assessment. Restraint use reduction is now an international issue with institutions working to decrease both restraint use and patient falls (Moore and Haralambous 2007).While learning about the craft of research, nurses should also remember that the profession brings a unique perspective to addressing issues of great importance to the individuals and families in our care. Box 1-1 discusses some nursing studies that have made a difference.

Nursing research helps to define professional practice. Nurses have sought to increase the credibility of their professional practice. Utilizing knowledge based on scientific findings gives nursing additional credibility. Nurses need to demonstrate research-based practices that result in improved outcomes and cost-effective care. For example, can nursing demonstrate science-based practices that might prevent a patient on a ventilator from catching pneumonia? Such practices save the patient from experiencing a critical complication, reduce the need for expensive therapies, and keep the patient from spending additional days in the intensive care unit. Nursing research also increases professional accountability for practice. It is difficult to defend nursing practices that are not grounded in science. Research provides a scientific rationale for nursing care measures.

Research issues are also of concern to the public. Consumers are concerned about research findings that affect their personal lives. For example, since publication of the 1999 Institute of Medicine (IOM) report entitled *To Err Is Human*, public interest in medical errors and safety has moved to the forefront. The popular press has embraced the topic of safety and includes releases on relevant safety research in health care. Note *Research in the News* which presents safety research regarding medication errors. Nurses

BOX 1-1 Nursing Studies That Have Made a Difference

- A study by Dr. Linda Aiken examined safe staffing levels for hospitalized patients, determining that patient well-being is related to the level of nurse staffing.
- Dr. Nancy Bergstrom studied an instrument to better assess pressure ulcers (bedsores) in patients in order to prevent pressure ulcer formation. Result: new clinical guidelines were written to prevent and treat pressure ulcers.
- Concerned about diabetes in adolescents, Dr. Margaret Grey studied an intervention—Coping Skills Training—to improve teen diabetic management through a comprehensive program that increased coping skills, communication, health behaviors, and conflict resolution.
- Dr. Joanne Harrell studied the effects of education and exercise programs to improve youth physical activities. These interventions reduced cardiovascular risk.
- Dr. Kate Lorig examined programs to promote self-management of arthritis sufferers. Program participants reported greater abilities to manage their arthritis, improved activity levels, and better general health.

Visit the National Institute for Nursing Research at "http://www.nih.gov/ninr/"www.nih.gov/ninr/ Click on *About NINR* and then click on and scroll through the mission and strategic plan; peruse. Note the *areas of research emphasis*. Try the link on *Nursing Research-Making a difference*. What does this say to you about how research can impact nursing practice?

(National Institute of Nursing Research [NINR] 2006)

Resource and Subject Matter

Research in the News

Study: Interrupting a Nurse Makes Medication Errors More Likely

BY KAREN PALLARITO,
HealthDay Reporter © 2010 HealthDay
News, April 26, 2010

Distracting an airline pilot during taxi takeoff or landing could lead to a critical error. Apparently the same is true of nurses who prepare and administer medication to hospital patients.

A new study shows that interrupting nurses while they're tending to patients' medications increases the chance of error. As the number of distractions increases, so do the number of errors and the risk to patient safety.

"We found that the more interruptions a nurse received while administering a drug to a specific patient, the greater the risk of a serious error occurring," said the study's lead author, Johanna I Westbrook, director of the Health Informatics Research and Evaluation Unit at the University of Sydney in Australia.

. . . For the study, the researchers observed 98 nurses preparing and administering 4,271 medications to 720 patients . . . Using handheld computers, the observers recorded the nursing procedures during medication administration, details of the medication administered, and the number of interruptions experienced.

continued . . .

. . . Only one in five drug administrations (19.8%) was completely error free, the study found.

Most errors were minor (79.3%), having little or no impact on patients, according to the study. However, 115 (2.7%) were considered major errors, and all of them were clinical errors.

. . . one potential remedy: A 'protected hour' during which nurses would focus on medication administration without having to do such things as take phone calls or answer pages.

. . . Not all interruptions are bad, West-brook added. "If you are being given a drug and you do not know what it is for, or you are uncertain about it, you should interrupt and question the nurse," she said.

Here is a report on a research study that made headline news.

> What useful practice messages come from this research study?
>
> How might nurses want to modify their clinical practice in order to protect patient safety?
>
> How do you think the public might respond to these findings?

The answers are there—here are key sentences regarding the findings:

interrupting nurses while they're tending to patients' medications increases the chance of error.

. . . Only one in five drug administrations (19.8%) was completely error free, the study found.

a "protected hour" during which nurses would focus on medication administration without having to do such things as take phone calls or answer pages.

Not all interruptions are bad, . . . "If you are being given a drug and you do not know what it is for , or you are uncertain about it, you should interrupt and question the nurse,"

Check out the actual research study at:

Westbrook, J., A. Woods, W. Dunsmuir, and R. Day. 2010. Association of interruptions with an increased risk and severity of medication administration errors. *Archives of Internal Medicine. 170*(8): 683–690.

have intuitively known that interruptions affect their concentration when they are giving medications. Here is evidence that is of vital interest to nurses and consumers alike.

History

Nursing research has a long and fruitful past. We are fortunate to have a rich history beginning in the 19th century with Florence Nightingale, the first nurse researcher. Nightingale's research skills included recording information, which she then organized and analyzed to draw conclusions about the effectiveness of nursing care (Dossey 2000). Nightingale was one of the first to present evidence with mathematical statistics, a cutting-edge endeavor during the 1800s. Her care and documentation of outcomes impacted practice because she was able to effectively communicate this information to others. Before arriving at a Crimean war hospital during the mid-1800s, the death rate at war front hospitals was 42.7%. Four times as many deaths were caused by disease as were caused by wounds. Attributing these deaths to poor sanitation, Nightingale implemented a program to improve cleanliness of patients and the facility. At the end of her tenure, the mortality rate had fallen to 2.2% (Dossey 2000). Her actions directly affected patient care as well as provided insight for policy initiatives that would facilitate care, both goals of nursing research. Following the war, she revolutionized hospital data collection and was responsible for developing the Uniform Hospital Discharge Data. This information linked mortality rates with diagnoses and treatments (Dossey 2000). Nightingale's work exemplifies the process of changing practice through nursing research.

When examining the history of nursing research, we find that nursing stands on the shoulders of those nurses who have gone before us. Successful nursing research depends not only on nurses who are actually conducting studies, but on many factors. Adequate education in research methods, financial support for research from private and government sources, and institutional support all influence the quality and quantity of nursing research. All of these factors have evolved over time.

Consider This . . .

Sir Isaac Newton famously said, "If I have seen further than others it is by standing on the shoulders of giants." What do you think he meant and how does this statement apply to nursing research?

Gortner (2000) divides historical development of nursing research into three phases: early years (from Nightingale through 1964), the transition years from 1965 to 1985 (when nursing research became nursing science), and a period from 1985 and beyond (when nursing science comes of age). Let us examine a few significant events in each of those phases.

Early Years

While Nightingale's strong research focus was an excellent start, nursing research evolved slowly. During the early years, nursing was gradually advancing as a profession through education and licensure. Concerns of nursing during this period were public health, communicable diseases of both children and adults, and maternal and child health (Gortner 2000). Nursing education programs steadily proliferated in the late 1800s after the first hospital-based school of nursing was established in 1872. As a mark of increasing professionalization, a journal dealing with nursing concerns, the *American Journal of Nursing,* was initiated in 1900. The first university-based nursing program began in 1909. In 1923, the Goldmark Report, describing deficiencies in nursing education and recommending advanced education for nursing educators and leaders, was published. It sometimes surprises people to learn that the first doctoral program for nurses was established in 1924 at Teachers College, Columbia. Early nursing research studies began in the 1920s dealing with issues such as hand washing, nursing care activities, and thermometer disinfection. A major step for nursing occurred in 1936 when the Honor Society for Nursing Sigma Theta Tau began funding nursing research.

During the years surrounding World War II in the 1940s, national data were collected on nursing needs and resource utilization (Gortner 2000). The Division of Nursing Resources was created as part of the Department of Public Health in 1948. This division became an important source of support for nursing research. Quality of nursing education remained a concern, which generated the 1948 Brown Report, a national study of nursing education which recommended moving nursing education to university settings. The report also recommended that nurse educators needed to be involved in nursing research.

Significant events occurred during the 1950s. *Nursing Research,* a journal devoted exclusively to research about nursing concerns, was first published in 1952. In 1955, the American Nurses Association (ANA) established the American Nurses Foundation to support programs of nursing excellence. Nursing research received another boost when the U.S. Public Health Service began funding nursing research grants and supporting nurse fellowship programs in 1955. Walter Reed Hospital established a unit devoted to nursing research in 1957. By the sixties, federal support was given to establish a Nurse Scientist Training Grant program to prepare nurses in basic science through the doctoral level. This additional educational preparation promoted development of many nurse scientists. At this point, information about available nursing literature—particularly research literature—was not located in a central index that facilitated gathering literature resources. Through the work of Virginia Henderson, the *Nursing Studies Index,* which compiled nursing research from 1900 through 1959, was published in 1963. This index represented the first organized listing of nursing research literature in one place.

Transition Years

From 1965 to 1985, nursing's influence increased in the federal policy arena with regard to nursing education and research (Gortner 2000). Increased funding for nursing education and research resulted. Education for nurses also moved to college- and university-based programs. Broad-based nursing theories were developed and dissemination of research findings became an emphasis. The ANA established the Council of Nurse Researchers in 1972, and there was an impetus to tie nursing research, particularly research supported by federal dollars, to health priorities. In 1974, the ANA designated research priorities for the next decade. By 1976, the ANA Commission on Nursing Research advocated for incorporating nursing research into nursing education programs and continuing education for practicing nurses. Additional research journals began during this period including *Research in Nursing and Health* (1978) and *Western Journal of Nursing Research* (1979). Advanced educational programs proliferated and more nurses began engaging in nursing research. Once again, in 1980, the ANA Cabinet on Nursing Research set research priorities for the coming decade. This document was followed in 1985 by a Cabinet of Nursing Research publication entitled *Directions for Nursing Research: Toward the Twenty-first Century.*

Significant nursing research studies emerged during this period that influenced not only nursing practice, but other disciplines as well (Donaldson 2000). For example, Jeanne Quint Benoliel used qualitative research techniques to study the experience of women following mastectomy; she found that not informing women of their breast cancer diagnosis had a negative impact on their patient experiences. Her findings helped to modify communication practices in serious illness.

Collecting data significant to nursing emerged as a primary concern during the 1990s. The ANA began to collect and evaluate information called nurse sensitive indicators. Nurse sensitive indicators reflect the level of nursing care and care outcomes directly related to nursing care such as falls, catheter associated urinary tract infections, central line infections, ventilator associated pneumonia, and pressure ulcers (NDNQI, 2011).

Age of Nursing Science

During this period a new maturity came to the world of nursing research due to the emergence of aggregate studies, additional numbers of doctorally prepared faculty with programs of research, the ability of faculty to direct their time and effort toward research, competitive research funding, substantive research activities, and the emergence of leadership that supported research (Gortner 2000). A significant event promoting the growth of the nursing research enterprise occurred when the National Center for Nursing Research (NCNR) was established at the National Institutes of Health (NIH) in 1986. This event provided additional sources for federal funding for research as well as providing a body to establish priorities for nursing research. In 1993, the NCNR became the National Institute of Nursing Research (NINR) giving the institute greater status in the NIH.

Several additional nursing research journals began, including *Qualitative Health Research,* in 1990. Nursing entered the digital age in 1993 with the *Online Journal of Knowledge Synthesis* begun by Sigma Theta Tau International—the Honor Society for Nursing. Publications focusing on evidence-based practice and embracing a global approach are now emerging. *WORLDviews on Evidence Based-Nursing* began in 2004 as a publication for synthesis of evidence, providing links to global evidence-based resources.

Two important reports influenced research trajectories in nursing. During 1999, the Institute of Medicine (IOM) published a report entitled *To Err Is Human: Building a Safer Health Care System.* The report called for establishing a national focus for leadership, research, tools, and protocols to improve safety. Impetus was given to developing better technology to reduce errors, focus on the effectiveness of safety interventions, focusing on safety through demonstration projects, utilizing multidisciplinary teams of researchers to find causes of errors and test solutions, and providing funding for safety research (IOM 1999). A decade later, a second groundbreaking report from the Robert Wood Johnson Foundation (2010) Initiative on the Future of Nursing at the IOM entitled *The Future of Nursing: Leading Change, Advancing Health* recommended doubling the number of nurses with doctoral degrees by 2020. It further indicated that nurses should practice to the full extent of their education and foster interprofessional collaboration by serving as full partners in health care redesign. Nursing research would clearly be a part of providing evidence for health care change.

As we continue to move ahead, a critical mass of nurses are doctorally prepared and strong impetus is present to increase those numbers. Nursing is embracing the electronic age—which increases the sophistication of data collection and the dissemination of critical research information. If carefully designed, use of electronic medical records has the potential to increase the number of data sources to evaluate nurse sensitive indicators about specific concerns such as pressure ulcers and falls. Partnering with other health care professionals in our research will become increasingly critical. Building on our history, we need to forge ahead to discover new information and work to apply significant findings to our practice. Check out Box 1-2 for a summary of historical points in nursing research.

BOX 1-2 Important Events in Nursing Research

Date	Event
Early Years—Nightingale to 1964	
Mid 1800s	Florence Nightingale: Crimean War care documentation, *Notes on Nursing,* Uniform Hospital Discharge Data
1872	The first U.S. hospital based nursing program was established.
1900	*American Journal of Nursing* first published
1909	First university nursing program established
1923	Goldmark Report on nursing education published
1924	First doctoral program for nursing began at Teachers College, Columbia
1920s	First nursing research studies emerge Case studies emerge as a teaching tool
1936	Nursing Honor Society Sigma Theta Tau funds research
1948	Division of Nursing Resources created Brown Report published
1952	*Nursing Research* first published
1955	American Nurses Foundation established to fund research U.S. Public Health Service funds nursing research
1957	Walter Reed Hospital establishes a unit for nursing research
1960	Faye Abdellah publishes 21 nursing problems which were research based
1963	*Nursing Studies Index* published by Virginia Henderson
Transition Years—1965 to 1985	
1972	American Nurses Association (ANA) establishes Council of Nurse Researchers
1974	ANA designates first set of research priorities
1976	ANA Commission on Nursing Research recommends research education
1978	*Research in Nursing and Health* first published
1985	ANA publishes *Directions for Nursing Research: Toward the Twenty-first Century*

Date	Event
Age of Nursing Science—1986 to present	
1986	National Center for Nursing Research (NCNR) established
1988	*Applied Nursing Research* first published
1989	Agency for Health Care Policy and Research (AHCPR) established (later renamed Agency for Healthcare Research and Quality [AHRQ]
	ANA publishes *Education for Participation in Nursing Research* (becomes position statement in 1994)
1990	*Qualitative Health Research* first published
1993	NCNR becomes National Institute of Nursing Research (NINR)
	Online *Journal of Knowledge Synthesis* first available
1998	American Association of Colleges of Nursing (AACN) approves position statement on nursing research
1999	Institute of Medicine (IOM) Report *To Err Is Human: Building a Safer Health Care System* provides impetus for research on safe care
2006	NINR identifies research priorities for 2006–2010
2010	*Healthy People 2020*, published by U.S. Department of Health and Human Services
2010	Report by the Robert Wood Johnson Foundation on the Future of Nursing at the IOM titled *The Future of Nursing: Leading Change, Advancing Health* calls for advancing levels of nursing education and assumption of partnership with other health care professionals to impact health care

Nursing Research Roles

All nurses have roles to play in nursing research. No nurse is exempt. At first glance, roles in nursing research are not necessarily discernable. After examination, however, research roles become more apparent. Roles are tied to education, as well as the processes on consuming findings, guiding the research process, and collaboration.

Research Roles Tied to Nursing Educational Levels

Educational preparation helps to determine research roles. Nurses with associate degrees, baccalaureate degrees, master's degrees, and doctoral degrees learn different skills that facilitate participation in research. The American Nurses Association Position Statement on *Education for Participation in Nursing Research* (1994) tied research roles that nurses might play to level of educational preparation. This paper differentiated the research focus for each level of nursing education to ensure that nurses were well grounded in their respective research roles. The paper affirmed that all nurses have a role in the nursing research enterprise (ANA 1994). Further, all nurses have a commitment to research and advancing the science of nursing. The ANA proposed that research education should be part of undergraduate education and continue to evolve throughout advanced education. The American Association of Colleges of Nursing (AACN) (2006a) has also suggested roles in nursing research tied to educational levels.

> **Consider This . . .**
>
> What role do you see yourself and your classmates playing in nursing research? How do your ideas match the roles described below?

ASSOCIATE DEGREE NURSES. The American Nurses Association Position Statement on *Education for Participation in Nursing Research* (1994) suggests that associate degree nurses are prepared to help identify clinical problems and assist with collection of data. While working in conjunction with nurses that hold more advanced credentials, associate degree nurses should use research findings for clinical care. For example, an associate degree nurse might identify safety concerns on a clinical unit as an area for further investigation and as part of a research team gather information regarding nurses' practices of checking patients' identification prior to medication administration.

BACCALAUREATE DEGREE NURSES. Baccalaureate nurses are also expected to identify clinical problems for research as well as help investigators gain clinical site access. Baccalaureate prepared nurses should also influence data collection methodologies for specific studies. In addition, baccalaureate prepared nurses have a role in reading and evaluating research for potential utilization in nursing practice (ANA 1994). According to the AACN, baccalaureate graduates should understand basic research processes and apply research findings as well as identify problems and collaborate on research teams. For example, a baccalaureate nurse might identify patient falls as a critical issue on the clinical unit. The nurse may be part of a team that reviews existing research on falls that subsequently devises a research-based plan to reduce the number of patient falls on the unit. The nurse then would be part of a systematic evaluation to see if the intervention to reduce falls was effective.

MASTER'S DEGREE NURSES. Nurses completing graduate programs have additional research responsibilities because of their advanced educational preparation. The ANA (1994) specifically identified nurses with a master's degree as clinical experts who are well prepared to serve as collaborators in nursing research, working with experienced investigators. Master's prepared clinicians are prepared to judge the relevance of research outcomes for clinical practice. Master's prepared administrators can facilitate the creation of a climate that supports inquiry and subsequent application of research findings in clinical practice. The AACN (2006a) suggests that master's prepared clinicians should be capable of evaluating research and developing and implementing practice-based guidelines. These nurses should serve as leaders in identifying clinical problems for study and collaborating with nurse scientists for research initiation.

DOCTORALLY PREPARED NURSES. The ANA position paper (1994) indicated that nurses with doctoral degrees received advanced training in research skills. Expectations for doctorally prepared nurses include identifying significant research problems and developing programs for research that will benefit patients and the profession of nursing. Further expectations for doctorally prepared nurses include having knowledge of theories about nursing and ethical research conduct, the ability to design sound studies and acquire funding, and disseminating findings following the completion of studies (ANA 1994). For completed research, doctorally prepared nurses are responsible for communicating the study findings. According to the AACN (2006a), research-focused doctoral graduates should pursue and serve as leaders in conducting research for knowledge extension.

Since the creation of the American Nurses Association position statement regarding nurses' roles in research, there is now another level of doctoral education for nurses engaged in clinical practice, the Doctor of Nursing Practice (DNP). The focus of DNP preparation is advanced clinical practice. The AACN (2006b) indicates that nurses with DNP preparation should engage in clinical scholarship and should critically appraise literature to ascertain best clinical practices. They are responsible for evaluating outcomes of practice, designing quality improvement studies, and using relevant research findings for developing practice guidelines (AACN 2006a, 2006b). Additionally, DNP-prepared nurses work in collaboration with others for research and dissemination.

Nurse Consumers: Using Research Findings

Just what is a **consumer of research**? A consumer is a person who uses research findings. In many instances nurses are the major consumers of nursing research. Associate degree and baccalaureate nurses are vital players in the process of using research findings in patient care. Important skills in the process are the ability to critically read research studies and to apply study findings in a patient care setting. In some workplaces nurses may have journal clubs where nurses get together for the purpose of reading and discussing completed research studies and the implications they have for practice.

Nurse Scientists: Initiate and Guide the Process

Nurse scientists are those nurses who possess the education to identify critical research problems, to plan research to further investigate the problem, and to complete the research study. Nurse scientists consist of nurses with a doctoral education that specifically develop their research skills. These nurses are key players in designing and securing funding to conduct the research. They are also key leaders in pulling together nursing teams for the conduct of research. Many institutions may have a nurse scientist whose role is to facilitate nursing research. These nurses may lead nursing research studies or work to facilitate nurses employed by the institution in their research efforts.

Nurse scientists need to establish programs of research consisting of multiple related studies about significant nursing problems. While single studies in an area of research is useful, programs of research add greater depth to nursing knowledge and have the potential for a larger impact on patient care.

Nurse Collaborators: Working with Others to Discover

Collaboration means that people work together in order to accomplish a common goal. Collaboration can take many different forms in nursing research. For example, nurses at many different educational levels can work on a research project together. Imagine a team composed of nurse scientists, bedside nurses, and clinical nurse experts.

We are at a critical phase in health care that requires nurses work with one another and with other disciplines to conduct research and implement processes to utilize research findings. **Multidisciplinary research**—research where nurses work with other health care disciplines—is becoming a more important process. Sometimes the term interdisciplinary research is used to describe multi-disciplinary research. A new initiative in the health care research world, **translational research,** focuses on moving research findings into practice (Woolf 2008). The NIH, an important source of federal funding for health care research, began this initiative to ensure that research findings made their way into clinical practice more rapidly. All translational research that is multidisciplinary offers nurses more opportunities to play a role on collaborative research teams comprised of many types of health care providers.

Evidence-Based Practice—Research in Action

Although the phrase evidence-based practice (EBP) sounds terribly formal, in practical terms evidence-based practice means applying research findings to clinical practice. Ingersoll (2000) defines **evidence-based practice** as "the conscientious, explicit and judicious use of theory-derived, research based information in making decisions about patient care delivery to individuals or groups of patients and in consideration of individual needs and preferences" (p. 152). Evidence-based practice serves as a mechanism for resolving clinical problems and promoting high quality care that meets the needs of patients and families (Melnyk and Fineout-Overholt 2010).

> **Consider This . . .**
>
> What impact, if any, do you think nursing research can have on nursing practice?

Many different types of research studies may be incorporated into evidence-based practice (Melnyk and Fineout-Overholt 2010). Say, for example, that you are caring for a patient with an ischemic stroke. How much should the head of the bed be elevated to ensure the best blood flow to the brain? Traditional practice dictated that the head of the bed should be elevated 30°. Nurse Anne Wojner (Wojner, El-Mitwalli, and Alexandrov 2002) studied the brain blood flow of ischemic stroke patients who were positioned with the head of their bed elevated at three different levels: 30°, 15°, and flat. Wojner found that ischemic stroke patients had increased blood flow to the brain with lower elevation levels, particularly with a flat position. Research such as this study provides evidence, along with other findings from the literature that can be used to change practice, thus promoting more effective patient care.

The evidenced-based practice movement began in medicine during the late 1970s. At that time, only a limited number of research findings made their way into clinical practice. Additionally, it took nurses a long time between completing research studies to implement their findings. EBP also supports the concept of systematically considering multiple studies as a basis for the evidence to change practice, a shift from utilizing single studies as sources of practice change. Evidence-based practice has extended from medicine to other areas in health care and to areas outside of the health care arena.

Evidence-based practice is more than reading some articles and deciding to try new ideas. Several steps are involved in the evidence-based practice process (Melnyk and Fineout-Overholt 2010):

- Ask the clinical question relevant to the problem to be solved or change considered.
- Search and collect evidence that will facilitate answering the question.
- Critically appraise the evidence to evaluate strengths and weaknesses.
- Implement the best evidence, if appraisal indicates sufficient evidence is present.
- Evaluate the outcome of the implementation to ensure the change is creating positive outcomes.

Chapters 9 and 10 present much more information about evidence-based practice and its implementation.

What Does the Future Hold?

While the future of nursing research is very bright, there is still much progress needed. The good news is that a substantial body of nursing research knowledge is bringing about practice changes. Nursing research continues to forge ahead and is often embedded into programs of research consisting of multiple studies that build on other related studies. Nursing still has many areas to research in the future and needs to work to ensure completed research is disseminated and utilized in practice. As a result, nursing must develop strategies to guide the nature of future research. Additionally, the nursing profession must work to facilitate further research through funding and by educating nurses to use and conduct definitive research.

Research Priorities

Many areas in nursing require further research. However, there are limits to the number of nurse scientists and the levels of funding for research. Because of these limitations, nurses must strategically plan how to focus research and develop priorities for the types of research to receive funding. This type of direction focuses our research to achieve the greatest impact despite resource limitations. Beginning in the seventies, the ANA established research priorities. Now, the NINR, a major funding agency for nursing research, has held several conferences of nursing scientists to identify priorities for nursing research.

The NINR published the most recent set of priorities for research emphasis in 2011. These areas include the following (NINR 2011; p. 7):

- Enhance health promotion and disease prevention
- Improve quality of life by managing symptoms of acute and chronic illness
- Improve palliative and end of life care
- Enhance innovation in science and practice
- Develop the next generation of nurse scientists

Other bodies also identify areas of concern for health care research. For example: *Healthy People 2020* is a document by the U.S. Department of Health and Human Services (2010) that designates specific targets for achievement in health outcomes. Although research goals are not specifically listed, the goals for improvements in health care outcomes offer guidance to priority areas for research. Safe models of health care that reduce errors continue to receive priority.

Facilitators and Barriers

Nursing practice is forging ahead with an increasing number of interventions based on science. Other disciplines have started to recognize the value of nursing research contributions. In her review of breakthroughs in nursing research, Donaldson (2000) noted nursing research studies that impacted other disciplines. For example, nurse researcher Jean Johnson demonstrated that people could rate their level of pain, thus impacting the way pain was assessed in clinical practice. Donaldson cites another example in the research of Brooton, Brown, and Sachs, who developed the site transitional care model to reduce risks for very low birth weight infants that were discharged early from hospitals. When supervised by a clinical nurse specialist, infants successfully transitioned to the community thereby reducing costs and preventing readmissions. This evidence-based model was later used in multidisciplinary settings. Nursing research is receiving greater support than ever before, and nurses are playing a greater role in multidisciplinary research. However, we still face barriers in our research enterprise. When reviewing the facilitators and barriers to nursing research and evidence-based practice, consistent concerns for nursing research include funding, education, and institutional support.

> ### Consider This . . .
>
> What do you see as the biggest barrier for nurses when it comes to using nursing research in their workplaces?

A number of facilitators propel nursing research forward. Nursing research relates to significant issues in health care such as an aging population, a shift in focus to prevention, and care for chronic conditions. Nurses have a strong history of concern in those areas and will be key players in the future. Educational preparation of nurses has improved. Almost 1% of all registered nurses have completed a doctoral degree (HRSA 2010). This means that the potential pool of nurse scientists is larger than ever before. As indicated by the Robert Wood Johnson (2010) report, double the number of doctorally prepared nurses are needed to meet future demands for research and education. Greater funding for research is available, although nursing still receives proportionally less than disciplines such as medicine. There is greater impetus for interdisciplinary research to improve safety (IOM 1999). Nursing has the opportunity for involvement in efforts to translate research findings into practice (MacGuire 2006).

Nursing research and EBP still face obstacles to success. Consistent barriers include negative attitudes about research, a knowledge gap about EBP (Melnyk et al. 2008), and organizational barriers such as a lack of time, limited access to resources, and weak institutional support (Hoss and Hanson 2008). In spite of the barriers, hope exists for strengthening our research practices. Strategies include:

1. Providing foundational educational programs for faculty as well as students to increase proficiency (Melnyk et al. 2008)
2. Reallocating institutional resources to support data gathering (Hoss and Hanson 2008)
3. Shifting institutional values (MacGuire 2006)
4. Initiating new knowledge discussion groups for students and staff nurses (Moch and Cronje 2007)
5. Incorporating EBP into practice standards (Resnick 2006)

Although significant barriers to research are present, nurses possess the strategic skills to move a research agenda forward, ensuring that important discoveries are made and incorporated into practice.

SUMMARY

The world of nursing research has exciting potential. Nurses need to embrace the process of research in terms of advancing our search for knowledge and in using our current knowledge to benefit the patients and families for whom we care. Here is a summary of key points in this chapter.

- Nurses have used many sources of information to guide practice, including **traditional practices, authority, personal experience, intuition, trial-and-error,** and **inductive** or **deductive reasoning.** *(Objective 1)*

- **Nursing research** allows for systematic discovery of information and the application of the information discovered to clinical practice, administration, or education. *(Objective 2)*

- The history of nursing research is rich in examples of how nursing has made strides toward a scientific knowledge base for practice. *(Objective 3)*

- Nursing research roles are tied to educational levels of nurses. All nurses have a role in nursing research. Nurses may be **consumers of research**, serve as **nurse scientists**, and collaborate with others to conduct and use both **multidisciplinary** and **translational** research. *(Objective 4)*

- **Evidence-based practice** is a method for applying research findings to clinical practice. Multidisciplinary research and evidence-based practice are a part of nursing's future. *(Objective 5)*

- Major organizations have identified research priorities in health care, including but not limited to promoting health, preventing disease, and eliminating disparities in access to care. *(Objective 6)*

- In spite of existing barriers to using nursing research, such as negative attitudes or lack of institutional support, nurses possess key skills to conduct research and incorporate findings into practice. *(Objective 7)*

Review the following questions, visit the web site, and work the web exercises designed for this chapter.

Resource and Subject Matter

STUDENT ACTIVITIES

Now it is time for you to see whether you can apply what you have learned.

1. List at least five reasons why nursing research is relevant to the practice of nursing.

2. Examine again the methods listed by which we learn. What are your predominant modes of gaining new knowledge?

3. Interview an RN. Ask if he/she makes use of research in his/her practice. If the answer is yes, ask follow-up questions to find out how. If not, explore why not.

4. Explore the institution where you are currently assigned for clinical practice. Does the institution promote evidence-based practice? In what ways do they make evidence-based practice a reality? In what ways could they do more?

Pearson Nursing Student Resources

Find additional review materials at
www.nursing.pearsonhighered.com
Prepare for success with additional NCLEX®-style practice questions, interactive assignments and activities, web links, animations and videos, and more!

REFERENCES

American Association of Colleges of Nursing (AACN). 2006a. *AACN position statement on nursing research*. Washington, DC: Author. Retrieved April 30, 2010. http://www.aacn.nche.edu/Publications/pdf/NsgResearch.pdf

American Association of Colleges of Nursing (AACN). 2006b. *The essentials of doctoral education for advanced nursing practice*. Washington, DC: Author. Retrieved April 30, 2010. http://www.aacn.nche.edu/DNP/pdf/Essentials.pdf

American Nurses Association (ANA). 1994. *Education for participation in nursing research*. Kansas City, MO: Author. http://www.nursingworld.org/MainMenuCategories/HealthcareandPolicyIssues/ANAPositionStatements/research/rseducat14484.aspx

American Nurses Association (ANA). 1985. *Directions for nursing research: Toward the twenty-first century*. Kansas City, MO: Author.

Benner, P. 1984. *From novice to expert: Excellence and power in clinical nursing practice*. Menlo Park, CA: Addison-Wesley.

Donaldson, S.K. 2000. Breakthroughs in scientific research: The discipline of nursing, 1960–1999. *Annual Review of Nursing Research, 18*: 247–311.

Dossey, B. 2000. *Florence Nightingale: Mystic, visionary, healer.* Springhouse, PA: Springhouse.

Gortner, S. 2000. Historical development in nursing: Our historical roots and future opportunities. *Nursing Outlook, 48*(2): 60–67.

Health Resources and Services Administration (HRSA). 2010. *The registered nurse population: Findings from the 2008 national sample survey of registered nurses*. http://bhpr.hrsa.gov/healthworkforce/rnsurveys/rnsurveyfinal.pdf

Hoss, B. and D. Hanson. 2008. Evaluating the evidence: Web sites. *AORN Journal, 87*(1): 124–141.

Ingersoll, G. 2000. Evidence-based nursing: What it is and what it isn't. *Nursing Outlook, 48*(4): 151–152.

Institute of Medicine (IOM). 1999. *To err is human: Building a safer health system*. Washington, DC: National Academies Press. http://www.nap.edu/openbook.php?isbn=0309068371

Lajiness, M., C. Wolfert, S. Hall, C. Sampselle, and A. Diokno. 2007. Group session teaching of behavioral modification program for urinary incontinence: Establishing the teachers. *Urologic Nursing, 27*(2): 124–127.

Langford, R. 2001. *Navigating the maze of nursing research*. St. Louis, MO: Mosby.

MacGuire, J. 2006. Putting nursing research findings into practice: Research utilization as an aspect of the management of change. *Journal of Advanced Nursing, 53*(1): 65–74.

Melnyk, B. and E. Fineout-Overholt. 2010. *Evidence-based practice in nursing and healthcare: A guide to best practice* (2nd ed.). Philadelphia, PA: Lippincott, Williams, and Wilkins.

Melnyk, B., E. Fineout-Overholt, N. Feinstein, L. Sadler, and C. Green-Hernandez. 2008. Nurse practitioner educators' perceived knowledge, beliefs, and teaching strategies regarding evidenced-based practice: Implications for accelerating the integration of evidenced-based practice into graduate programs. *Journal of Professional Nursing, 24*(1): 7–13.

Moch, S. and R. Cronje. 2007. New knowledge discussion groups: Counteracting the common barriers to evidence-based practice. *WORLDviews on Evidence-Based Nursing, 4*: 112–115.

Moore, K. and B. Haralambous. 2007. Barriers to reducing the use of restraints in residential elder care facilities. *Journal of Advanced Nursing, 58*(6): 532–540. doi 10.1111/j.1365-2648.2007.04298.x

National Institute of Nursing Research (NINR). 2006. *Changing practice, changing lives: 10 landmark nursing research studies* (Pub No. 06-6094). Retrieved from the National Institutes of Health, National Institute of Nursing Research. Retrieved October 30, 2008. http://www.ninr.nih.gov/NR/rdonlyres/27F3FB10-FE62-4119-9FA9-1140B6950AFF/0/10LandmarkNursingResearchStudies508.pdf

National Institute of Nursing Research (NINR). 2011. *Bringing science to life: NINR strategic plan* (Pub No. 11-7783). Retrieved March 12, 2012 from the National Institutes of Health, National Institute of Nursing Research. http://www.ninr.nih.gov/AboutNINR/NINRMissionandStrategicPlan/

NDNQI. 2011. *NDNQI Transforming data into quality care*. Retrieved from https://www.nursingquality.org/

Pallarito, K. 2010. Interrupting a nurse makes medication errors more likely. *Health Day: News for Healthier Living*. http://www.healthday.com/Article.asp?AID=638474

Resnick, B. 2006. Outcomes research: You do have the time! *Journal of the American Academy of Nurse Practitioners, 18*: 505–509.

Robert Wood Johnson Foundation. 2010. *The future of nursing: Leading change, advancing health*. Washington, DC: National Academies Press. http://www.nap.edu/catalog/12956.html

Strumpf, N. and L. Evans. 1988. Physical restraint of the hospitalized elderly: Perceptions of patients and nurses. *Nursing Research, 37*: 132–137.

US Department of Health and Human Services (USDHHS). 2010. *Healthy people 2020: Understanding and improving health*. http://www.healthypeople.gov/document/

Winston, P., P. Morelli, J. Bramble, A. Friday, and J. Sanders. 1999. Improving patient care through implementation of nurse-driven restraint protocols. *Journal of Nursing Care Quality, 13*(6): 32–46.

Wojner, A., A. El-Mitwalli, and A. Alexandrov. 2002. Effect of head positioning on intracranial blood flow velocities in acute, ischemic stroke: A pilot study. *Critical Care Nursing Quarterly, 24*(4): 57–66.

Woolf, S. 2008. The meaning of translational research and why it matters. *Journal of the American Medical Association, 299*(2): 211–213.

Conducting Effective Searches for Evidence

CHAPTER OUTLINE

CHAPTER OBJECTIVES

1. Describe key components necessary for information retrieval.
2. Identify key databases available to access health care literature.
3. Discuss useful search strategies for perusing electronic databases.
4. Identify and describe selected nursing research and evidence-based resources.

KEY TERMS

Abstract **(p. 24)**

Bibliographic database
 (p. 24)

Boolean operators **(p. 29)**

CINAHL **(p. 24)**

Citation **(p. 24)**

Cochrane Collaboration
 (p. 25)

Database **(p. 23)**

Electronic database **(p. 24)**

Full text **(p. 24)**

MEDLINE **(p. 24)**

Periodical **(p. 24)**

Search **(p. 23)**

Search limits **(p. 29)**

Search parameters **(p. 27)**

Systematic review **(p. 25)**

ABSTRACT

Finding and using evidence that supports the use of the best nursing practices depends heavily on the ability to successfully retrieve pertinent resources through the skillful use of search techniques and appropriate databases. Research studies and systematic reviews in published journals provide the best resources for up-to-date objective evidence to guide practice. This chapter provides information retrieval mechanisms and processes and discusses leading published nursing research resources.

The purpose of this chapter is to help you find and retrieve the research and other evidence-based resources that are required for you to locate the best available evidence for your nursing practice. We will discuss databases and periodicals and examine strategies for effectively searching those databases to access and retrieve relevant journal articles.

Information Retrieval

The process of conducting a **search** to access and retrieve information has changed dramatically in the last decade, as a visit to a modern library makes clear. The process of using a library and performing a search of the literature has evolved. No longer do you have to manually search through card catalogs and large volumes of print indexes to find what you need. The entire process is computerized. The information to be searched is located in large electronic databases and most libraries subscribe to multiple databases. Articles in most mainstream periodicals are available electronically. You may not even need a physical visit to the library as most libraries allow remote access to their databases and periodicals over the Internet.

A **database** is a collected listing of related information. These databases are used in the scientific and academic communities but are also seen in social, business, and other everyday settings. These databases can cover anything from a listing of books, journal articles, or art to a listing of social networks, blogs, or shoe styles. There are even databases that compile lists of other databases.

Libraries employ what are known as **bibliographic databases**. These databases typically contain listings and information for printed and published materials. The most familiar examples include a catalog of books or an index of periodicals. The listing is usually in the form of a citation and may include an abstract of the material cited. A **citation** provides information that makes it easy to locate the material or reference cited. For example, when looking at a database that references journal articles, you will see a citation containing the author's name, the title of the article, the journal name, the volume number, and the year of publication.

Citations of books include the author, book title, publisher's name and geographic location, year of publication, and International Standard Book Number (ISBN). An ISBN is a unique numerical code that identifies each published book. Sometimes, databases include an abstract of the cited article. An **abstract** is simply a short summary of the article and can be useful for determining whether a particular article is relevant for your needs. You have an excellent example of the use of abstracts in this textbook, as one is contained at the beginning of each chapter.

Bibliographic databases may contain a broad collection of citations for published resources across academic and scientific disciplines, or more specialized collections that target a specific discipline or specialty. Most of these databases are fully computer-accessible and are thus also known as **electronic databases**. There are a large variety of these databases that cover a wide range of subjects and the number grows daily. Established electronic databases are typically available through commercial information retrieval services such as Cambridge Scientific Abstracts (CSA), Ebscohost (EBSCO), OVID, or ProQuest. Libraries contract through these commercial vendors and subscribe to a specified collection of electronic databases. The libraries then provide library users with access to these databases. If the library has remote access capabilities, you as a library patron can access and search the databases over the Internet.

> **Consider This . . .**
>
> Check with your academic library. What electronic databases are available? Do you have online access to the databases from your home computer?

Databases for Healthcare Literature

Two comprehensive databases serve as the major search tools for materials in nursing and health-related disciplines. They are the Cumulative Index to Nursing and Allied Health Literature (**CINAHL**) and Medical literature online (**MEDLINE**). The *CINAHL* database is a particularly important database for nurses and nursing. *CINAHL* is owned and operated by EBSCO and offers four versions of its database, including two that contain full text access for articles in many of the journals listed. **Full text** means that the entire article is available electronically. The basic *CINAHL* database provides indexing for more than 3,000 **periodicals** (also referred to as journals) in nursing and 17 allied health disciplines and contains more than a million records from 1981 to the present (http://www.ebscohost. com /cinahl/). It lists all applicable English-language nursing journals plus publications from the National League for Nursing (NLN) and the American Nurses Association (ANA). *CINAHL* also offers access to books on healthcare, conference proceedings, standards of practice, nursing dissertations, and selected software. The full text version of *CINAHL* adds full text options for 600 selected journals. An enhanced version of *CINAHL* known as *CINAHL Plus* provides indexing for an additional 1,000 journals dating back as far as 1937. The full text version provides full text access to more than 750 journals and 220 books and monographs. All four available versions provide abstracts for most citations generated by professional abstract writers (http://www.ebscohost.com/cinahl/).

The MEDLINE database was developed by the National Library of Medicine (NLM) and is available through NLM as well as commercial vendors including CSA, EBSCO, and OVID. NLM offers a free version known as PubMed that can be accessed via the Internet by entering "PubMed" into an Internet search engine. MEDLINE is well known as the foremost source for materials. The MEDLINE database contains more than 20 million indexed citations from over 5,000 journals in medicine, nursing, dentistry, veterinary medicine, allied health, and preclinical sciences dating as far back as 1950. Author-generated abstracts are available for articles in most of these journals (http://www.ncbi .nlm.nih.gov/pubmed/). MEDLINE, also available through EBSCO, contains access to full text articles for close to 1,500 journals dating back to 1965.

Another extremely useful database set for evidence-based health care literature is the Cochrane Database of Systematic Reviews (CDSR) and Database of Abstracts of Reviews of Effectiveness (DARE) (http://www.cochrane.org/). The CDSR and DARE were developed and are maintained by the **Cochrane Collaboration**. The Cochrane Collaboration is an international organization whose primary aim is to provide evidence that can be used to make well-informed decisions about the efficacy of health care interventions. The CDSR contains citations and abstracts for over 5,500 systematic reviews conducted by a Cochrane Collaboration review group and relates to a wide variety of health care interventions (http://www.cochrane.org/). A **systematic review** is a literature review that uses a precise method to search for and analyze findings from a number of research studies. These findings are then synthesized and summarized. Chapter 9 explores systematic reviews in more depth.

Consider This ...

Why might systematic reviews be considered a crucial tool in evidence-based practice?

Plain language summaries are also available for many of the database entries. DARE lists over 3,000 citations, abstracts, and summaries of systematic reviews that were carried out by other individuals or groups and which have been assessed for quality by Cochrane (http://www.cochrane.org/). Access to CDSR and DARE are free through the Cochrane website. To locate the site, just enter the term "Cochrane library" into an Internet search engine. The two databases are also available through commercial vendors such as EBSCO and OVID. Access to the full text reviews is available from any of the sources for a fee or through any library holding a subscription to the Cochrane collection.

Box 2-1 lists and describes some other databases you might find useful. These databases cover health care and related disciplines. The title of the database often describes its contents.

You can imagine how useful these electronic databases will be as you search for evidence to determine the efficacy of selected nursing interventions. Computerized databases provide you with flexible, time efficient, and powerful tools to conduct comprehensive searches on the topic(s) of your choosing. However, before you begin your search, it helps to have an organized plan or strategy. This is particularly useful if you are using multiple databases for your search.

BOX 2-1 Additional Bibliographic Databases

Alt Health Watch—This database focuses on complementary, holistic, and integrated approaches to health care and wellness. It offers abstracts and full text articles for more than 180 international journals and reports dating as far back as 1984, as well as access to alternative health-related pamphlets, booklets, book excerpts, and research.

Dissertation Abstracts—This database provides an index for every doctoral dissertation from all accredited Universities in the U.S. dating from 1861 and selected theses dating from 1988. Abstracts are available for all dissertation entries starting in 1980. It also includes selected theses and dissertations from Canada and Europe.

Educational Resources Information Center (ERIC)—The aim of this database is to provide access to a wide variety of education literature. ERIC is sponsored by the U.S. Department of Education and provides information about diverse materials such as books and monographs, reports and conference proceedings, theses and dissertations, government documents and directories, and registries. Listings start in1966.

LexisNexis Academic—This database contains access to citations, abstracts, and full text resources from diverse materials including magazines, newspapers, wire services, and government regulations and statutes for reference, business, health care, and legal disciplines. It is a comprehensive resource to research the current news available on a myriad of topics.

Psychology Information (PsychINFO)—This database provides citations with abstracts for literature in the psychological, social, behavioral, and health sciences. Included are over 2,000 journals and books dating from 1981.

Sociological Abstracts—This database provides indexes and abstracts for over 1,800 international journals in sociology and related disciplines in the social and behavioral sciences. It also provides abstracts of books, book chapters, dissertations, and conference papers. The citations date back to 1952.

Social Work Abstracts—This database provides indexes and abstracts for more than 450 journals in the social work and human services disciplines. Citations date back to 1977.

Web of Science—A compilation of citations from a number of multidisciplinary databases that provides a comprehensive integrated search platform for over 9,300 international research journals from 256 categories in the sciences (including medicine, nursing, and other health sciences), social sciences, arts, and humanities disciplines. This resource is maintained by the Institute for Scientific Information and includes the Science Citation Index, Social Sciences Index, Arts and Humanities Index, Index Chemicus, and Current Chemical Reactions.

Summaries accessed from http://www.ebscohost.com/

Search Strategies

This section is designed to help you make your searches smoother and more productive. There are several steps that you can employ to ensure a successful search.

- Define and refine topic
- Select appropriate resources
- Choose appropriate databases

- Define search parameters
- Run search
- Examine search results
- Collect resources from search

Define and Refine Topic

Before you run a search on any topic, you need to define and refine your topic. This will help you set **search parameters** to guide and focus your search. This means that you need to familiarize yourself with the major ideas and key concepts associated with that topic. If you already know precisely what you wish to search, this step is easy: just list your key terms and you are ready to move to the next step. However, if you have a more general subject idea, this step is vital to help you narrow the parameters of the search. Ask yourself the following questions: What is your subject area? What are key concepts and sub-concepts for that subject? What population are you interested in? Which concepts are most important? What information do you already have? Check out articles and reference books and Internet resources that you have access to. What kind of terms do they use when they describe your topic? Make a list of key concepts. Then list key words that typically describe each of these concepts. They can help focus and direct your search.

Say you were interested in bed sores in patients. Some preliminary investigation would lead you to use the correct subject heading *pressure ulcer*. Your population at this point is patients. You need to narrow your topic by identifying your area of interest. Are you searching for risk factors? Prevention? Assessment? Evaluation? Intervention? Treatment? Treatment types? Effectiveness of a specific intervention? The more concisely you can define and refine the search topic, the more productive your search will be. Suppose you decide that you want to know what will help prevent pressure ulcers in hospitalized adult patients. Your key concepts are pressure ulcers and prevention for a specified population of patients, namely adults who are hospitalized. Now you have a more refined topic that will lend itself more readily to a search.

Select Appropriate Resources

In this age of the information revolution, you as a nurse have access to an overabundance of available published literature relating to nursing and clinical practice. Entering any topic in your Internet search engine will confirm that. For example, I entered the term *pressure ulcers* in a popular computer search engine and got 880,000 results. These results included such entries as advertisements, books, articles, images, dictionaries, encyclopedias, PowerPoint slides, demonstrations, tutorials, and blogs. Even if you limit your search to the professional literature you will find books, journals, booklets, monographs, pamphlets, conference proceedings, and other miscellaneous publications. Thus choosing the most appropriate resources for your search really matters! Books tend to give you standard accepted information and practices. They provide good baseline data on a subject and can help you refine your search topic. Dictionaries, encyclopedias, booklets, and pamphlets are also good resources for quick definitions and overviews of your subject matter. Professional journals, on the other hand, provide information that is more current than that found in books. Journals report changing trends and practices. Research journals, in particular, are useful as they provide the results of the latest research investigations on your selected topic. These serve as key resources when you want to find the best evidence to guide your clinical practice.

> **Consider This ...**
>
> Why do you think research journals might be a key resource for locating evidence of the best way to provide nursing care?

Choose Appropriate Databases

When skimming a list of periodical indexes available from your library, some choices are obvious. You don't look in the literature or philosophy indexes for a nursing topic. However, as described earlier in this chapter, there are several indexes available for searching the health care literature and related disciplines. *CINAHL* and MEDLINE are the two best databases for comprehensive searches of health care literature. You might ask which is the better database to use? The answer depends on your subject of interest. *CINAHL* covers nursing, allied health, and psychosocial issues more comprehensively than MEDLINE, while MEDLINE offers much greater coverage of medicine and medical specialty. Most major nursing journals can be found in either index. It is often helpful to run a search using both databases.

Databases from other disciplines are often the best source when searching for information about a related topic in nursing. For example, you might locate articles for case management in the Social Work Abstracts. The most current information about effective educational strategies might be found in ERIC. Each database has a primary area of focus and has advantages and limits. The database's home page usually provides a description of its purpose and scope. You saw a quick summary for several of these databases in Box 2-1. Reading these descriptions can often help you decide which database might prove useful in a particular search.

Define Search Parameters

Once you have refined your topic, determined the type of resources needed, and selected a database, you need to set up the parameters for your search. You can search for keywords or combinations of words in any part of the article. You can do a cross search by entering several terms at once and instructing the computer on how to use those terms. You can place limits on the search by instructing the database to look only for certain groups of articles or certain types of journals or certain publication dates. After you enter the parameters, the search results appear with the touch of a button. If the search results are too vast or too scant, you can change the limits or keywords and instantly rerun your search.

When you open your selected database, you will be confronted with a search screen. The search mechanisms for each database operate in a slightly different fashion. In fact, the search mechanism can vary from vendor to vendor for the same database. For example, the search procedure mechanism for the MEDLINE database varies widely among the numerous vendors. The introductory computer screen and help feature that all the databases include will guide you in your search. Some database sites even provide quick tutorials on how to conduct searches on that site. Reference librarians can also be a great source of information and assistance.

Most basic searches usually begin by selecting and placing keywords in the search box. These are the major concepts that you identified in step one. Most databases will help you identify the preferred terms to use in your search. They will also let you view the entire directory of subjects and terms available if you are interested in how the database is organized. MEDLINE uses a medical subject-heading (MeSH) directory to index its articles. *CINAHL* uses its own specialized directory of subject headings as well. While there is some overlap in MEDLINE's and *CINAHL*'s subject headings, they are not the same. The varied subject headings allow you to retrieve information that may use different terminology for the same concept.

Let's look at sample results from an initial search using our example of preventing pressure ulcers in immobilized patients. We used the MEDLINE and *CINAHL* databases so you can compare them. The EBSCO host version 2.0 of both databases was used because the search mechanisms in all their database products have been totally revamped so that their databases use the same search mechanisms. The search mechanism itself has been greatly streamlined and simplified making it much easier and faster to use. Let's start by entering the term *pressure ulcer* into the search box. This results in 5,992 hits in *CINAHL* and 7,743 hits in MEDLINE. Checking so many citations for relevance would be unmanageable. So the search needs to be narrowed. That can done by adding terms to the search and by applying limits to the search.

To add search terms, let's use something called **Boolean operators**. These operators are just words (e.g., AND, OR) that help you to link key terms together to get certain results. Look at the terms *pressure ulcer* and *prevention* in Table 2-1. As you can see, OR is the least restrictive link and AND is the most restrictive link. In this case we want to use AND. So let's add *prevention* and link it to *pressure ulcer* with an AND. This results in 2,940 hits in *CINAHL* and 3,624 in MEDLINE. This is still too many citations to manage.

Let's place some search limits on the search. Some databases allow you to place **search limits** such as the age or gender of the population of interest, the language of the citations, publication types, journal types or specified journals, availability of an abstract, availability of full text, availability of references, and the date of publication for the articles. Not all limits are available in all databases. The databases allow you to easily add limits to further restrict citations or to lift limits if your search results become too restricted. For our example, let's choose the following limits: those entries for adult humans from research journals in English, with available abstracts from 2003 through 2008.

▶ Table 2-1 Boolean Operator Examples

Operator	Example	What Happens
OR	Pressure Ulcer **OR** Prevention	Retrieves all citations containing the words *pressure ulcer* OR the word *prevention*.
AND	Pressure Ulcer **AND** Prevention	Retrieves all citations containing the words *pressure ulcer* AND the word *prevention*.
NOT	Pressure Ulcer **NOT** Prevention	Retrieves all citations containing the words *pressure ulcer* except those with the word *prevention*.

▶ **Table 2-2   Search Limits**

Key Words/Limits	CINAHL Hits	MEDLINE Hits
Pressure Ulcer	5,992	7,743
Prevention	2,940	3,624
Humans	N/A	3,477
Adults	817	1,240
English only	770	1,014
Available abstract	557	709
2003 to 2008	258	254
Research Journals	179	136*

*MEDLINE has no limit for research journals so the limit of "Nursing journals" was applied.

Table 2-2 illustrates how the number of articles decreases with the addition of each limit. Now we have a workable number of citations.

It is helpful to keep a written record of the search terms and limits that you have chosen to enter. As you add new terms or limits, include them in your list. This provides a useful trail of your search should you wish to revisit the results at a future date.

The best way to become proficient at using database search techniques is through informed practice. Read the materials available on conducting a search. Use the help link on the database site or ask for assistance from a librarian if you aren't finding anything or if you are finding too much. Explore various search options and see what happens. With electronic databases, it is easy to try out various combinations of key terms and limits.

Run the Search

Once you have your terms and limits in place, it is easy to run your search. You just hit the search button and the list of citations will appear on the screen. A quick glance at the number of listed citations will let you know if you need to further limit the search or if you need to remove limits.

Examine Search Results

Once you have defined and run your search, you'll want to view the results. The results screen usually contains each citation in brief form with the option to view a full citation, an abstract, or full text when available. The EBSCO databases also use a technique called probabilistic searching. When a set of search terms and limits is entered and a search is run, the search results are rated by the relevancy of the citations and listed starting with the most relevant. Thus you see the most relevant article first. Figure 2-1 shows you an example of a brief citation as listed in the *CINAHL* database. A click on the title immediately brings up the full citation (see Figure 2-2). When you roll your cursor over on the magnifying glass, you are provided a pop-up screen with a view of the abstract. The pop-up disappears when you move your cursor. Note that this database also allows you to store this citation in a temporary folder. This is useful when making decisions about the

Research comparing three heel ulcer-prevention devices. 🔎
(includes abstract); Gilcreast DM; Warren JB; Yoder LH; Clark JJ;
Wilson JA; Mays MZ; Doughty D Journal of Wound, Ostomy &
Continence Nursing, 2005 Mar-Apr; 32 (2): 112-20 (journal article -
pictorial, *research*, tables/charts) ISSN: 1071-5754 PMID: 15867701
CINAHL AN: 2005075447
Abstract Only
⬜Add to folder | Relevancy: ▪▪▪▪▪▪▪ | Cited References: (27)
📄 PDF Full Text

■ **FIGURE 2-1** Sample Brief Citation from *CINAHL*
(http://www.ebscohost.com/cinahl/).

citations. There is a link to all published resources that have cited this particular study in
their publication and a link to the full text of the article. You can use this information to
help you determine the importance of the information in the article.

Examining the citations helps you determine which articles to keep and which to
eliminate because they are not relevant to your area of interest. Simply looking at article
titles can help you start this process. Some titles are clearly relevant and others obvi-
ously aren't. A third category may include citations that look feasible, yet the title does
not contain enough information to make a decision. If the citation looks promising, you
can instantly check the abstract for additional information by rolling over the magnifying
glass icon. If you decide to keep the article, add it to your temporary folder. As you work
your way through all the citations in your search, you will eventually fill your folder with
all the articles that you wish to keep.

Let's use the search on pressure ulcer prevention as an example. When viewing the
179 citations from the *CINAHL* search, the titles of 16 citations were clearly on target
so we placed them in a folder. The titles of 37 citations warranted further investigation so we examined the abstracts to determine their applicability. After viewing the
abstracts, we deemed 12 articles useful and added them to the folder. Titles in all other
citations clearly revealed that the articles were not useful to the investigation so we
marked them for elimination. In all, our search netted 28 useful articles on pressure
ulcer prevention. The citation results from the MEDLINE search were very similar and
netted many of the same articles.

Box 2-2 illustrates some examples from each decision category. Articles were placed
in various categories using several factors. You will note that each sample marked to keep
described a specific intervention for prevention. Some targeted for elimination discussed
specific populations such as spinal cord or HIV patients, focused on special settings such
as the operating room, or were only marginally related to the area of interest such as the
articles looking at nursing knowledge, testing the effectiveness of an instrument, or analyzing the economic impact of pressure ulcer treatment.

The titles warranting a closer look didn't have enough information in the title to
make a judgment. When viewing the abstract the choice became much easier. For example, in the article entitled *Preventing hospital-acquired pressure ulcers: a point prevalence study,* the abstract read in part "A cross-sectional study was conducted to ascertain
the effect of implementing a new support surface on the development of pressure ulcers
in one acute care facility" (Stewart et al. 2004). This description allows a reclassifica-
tion of this article as one to keep. The abstract from the article entitled *Measuring tissue*

> **BOX 2-2** Sample Titles from Pressure Ulcer Search Categorized by Determination of Usefulness
>
> **Titles of citations to keep**
> - Factors associated with pressure ulcers in adults in acute care hospitals.
> - Effectiveness of an alternating pressure air mattress for the prevention of pressure ulcers.
> - Physiological response of the heel tissue on pressure relief between three alternating pressure air mattresses.
> - Research comparing three heel ulcer-prevention devices.
> - Effectiveness of turning with unequal time intervals on the incidence of pressure ulcer lesions.
> - Reducing the incidence of pressure ulcers: implementation of a turn-team nursing program.
>
> **Titles warranting further investigation**
> - Guideline implementation results in a decrease of pressure ulcer incidence in critically ill patients.
> - Preventing hospital-acquired pressure ulcers: a point prevalence study.
> - Non-blanchable erythema as an indicator for the need for pressure ulcer prevention: a randomized-controlled trial.
> - Measuring tissue perfusion during pressure relief maneuvers: insights into preventing pressure ulcers.
> - Prevention of pressure ulcers in patients being managed on CLRT: is supplemental repositioning needed?
> - Continuous lateral rotation therapy.
> - Assessment of the cost of pressure sores treatment.
>
> **Titles of citations to eliminate**
> - A 4-cm thermo active viscoelastic foam pad on the operating room table to prevent pressure ulcer during cardiac surgery.
> - Patterns of recurrent pressure ulcers after spinal cord injury: identification of risk and protective factors 5 or more years after onset.
> - Incidence and risk factors associated with pressure ulcers among patients with HIV infection.
> - Intensive care nurses' knowledge of pressure ulcers: development of an assessment tool.
> - The prevalence of pressure ulcers in a tertiary care pediatric and adult hospital and effect of an educational program.
> - Inter-rater reliability of the EPUAP pressure ulcer classification system using photographs.
> - Modeling the economic losses from pressure ulcers among hospitalized patients in Australia.

perfusion during pressure relief maneuvers: insights into preventing pressure ulcers read in part "To study the effect on tissue perfusion of relieving interface pressure using standard wheelchair pushups compared with a mechanical automated dynamic pressure relief system. . . . Twenty individuals with motor-complete paraplegia below T4, 20 with motor-complete tetraplegia, and 20 able-bodied subjects. . ." (Makhsous et al. 2007). In this instance, the abstract helps eliminate the article because the article is discussing a specialized spinal cord injury population.

You can repeat the search steps for all relevant databases. In our example with pressure ulcers, for instance, it might be useful to run a search of the Cochrane databases to see if there are any systematic literature reviews on pressure ulcer prevention. A quick search using the terms *pressure ulcer* and *prevention* netted the following useful reviews: *Support surfaces for pressure ulcer prevention* published in 2008 and *Re-positioning for pressure ulcer prevention* published in 2003.

Looking at the citations may also give you clues about how to narrow your search. For example, there were a number of articles on spinal cord-injured patients in our pressure ulcer example. We were not interested in this specialized population. It would be useful to add spinal cord injury to the search terms using a Boolean operator NOT—so that articles about pressure ulcers in spinal cord injuries would be eliminated.

Viewing the full citation of an article can also be useful. In Figure 2-2, you will note direct links to the authors, the journal, related subject headings, and major subjects. A click on an author provides you with a list of other publications by that author. This can be useful in finding additional materials related to the topic. The journal link takes you to the electronic journal. The subject links take you to citations for those subject headings and may cue you to additional search avenues.

Collect Resources from Search

Once you have determined which articles meet your criteria, you need to locate a full copy of each one. Most major journals provide electronic copies of articles in full-text versions. These are free through subscription services at any academic library. They may also be purchased from the publishers or commercial vendors, who will e-mail them directly to your desktop. As you retrieve these articles, you need to determine how you wish to store, organize, and access them. Some people prefer to read hard copies of articles and thus choose to print out all the electronically retrieved articles. Others prefer to store and read the articles on their computer. Whatever your preference, you need an organizing system.

You might choose to store them by publication date or article title or journal of origin. A particularly useful organization strategy is to set up categories of focus. For example, our pressure ulcer articles might be organized into three major categories. One would include articles focusing on pressure ulcer risk factors. A second category would have articles discussing general or global approaches to prevention such as staff education or ulcer teams or institutional benchmarks. A third category could be used to file all articles that test an intervention, with subcategories established for each specific intervention (e.g., sub-files for articles on heel protectors, or turning, or mattress overlays).

Once you have obtained copies of all the articles, you can use the reference lists from the studies to conduct a secondary search. By reviewing the reference lists, you may find earlier research studies on your topic that could prove useful. When your articles are in electronic form, this task is often made easier as many electronic copies of articles now provide direct links to some of the articles in the reference list. You may also do a secondary search by examining other resources which have used and cited the articles that you have located. This has also been made easier in a number of databases. Refer again to Figure 2-1 on page 31. If you hit the Cited References link, it will instantly provide you with a list of the 27 sources that have cited this article in their publications. You can then determine if any of those materials look useful for your topic.

Title:	**Research comparing three heel ulcer-prevention devices.**
Authors:	Gilcreast DM; Warren JB; Yoder LH; Clark JJ; Wilson JA; Mays MZ
Affiliation:	Assistant Professor, University of Texas Health Science Center at San Antonio, dgilcreast@satx.rr.com
Editors:	Doughty D
Source:	Journal of Wound, Ostomy & Continence Nursing (J WOCN), 2005 Mar-Apr; 32(2): 112-20 (27 ref)
Publication Type:	Journal article - pictorial, *research*, tables/charts
Language:	*English*
Major Subjects:	Heel Pillows and Cushions -- Evaluation Pressure Ulcer -- Prevention and Control
Minor Subjects:	Adolescence; Adult; Aged; Aged, 80 and Over; Braden Scale for Predicting Pressure Sore Risk; Chi Square Test; Clinical Assessment Tools; Cost Benefit Analysis; Equipment Design; Female; Funding Source; Hospitals, Military; Incidence; Interrater Reliability; Male; Middle Age; Odds Ratio; Pillows and Cushions -- Economics; Post Hoc Analysis; Power Analysis; Pressure Ulcer -- Classification; Pressure Ulcer -- Epidemiology -- Texas; Pressure Ulcer -- Risk Factors; Prospective Studies; Quasi-Experimental Studies; Random Assignment; Texas
Abstract:	OBJECTIVE: To compare 3 *pressure*-reduction devices for effectiveness in *prevention* of heel ulcers in moderate-risk to high-risk patients. DESIGN: A prospective quasi-experimental 3-group design was used. SETTING AND SUBJECTS: A sample of 338 "moderate-risk to high-risk" *adult* inpatients, ages 18 to 97, at 2 medical centers in South Texas were studied. INSTRUMENTS: The Braden Scale for *Pressure Ulcer* Risk and investigator-developed history and skin assessment tools were used. METHODS: Subjects were randomly assigned to the High-Cushion Kodel Heel Protector (bunny boot), Egg Crate Heel Lift Positioner (egg crate), or EHOB Foot Waffle Air Cushion (foot waffle). Data are demographics, Braden scores, comorbidities, skin assessments, lengths of stay, and costs of devices. Analyses were Chi-square, analysis of variance, and regression. RESULTS: Of 240 subjects with complete data, 77 (32%) were assigned to the bunny boot group, 87 (36.3%) to the egg crate, and 76 (31.7%) to the foot waffle. Twelve ulcers developed in 240 subjects (5% incidence). Six subjects had only 1 foot. Eleven ulcers were Stage I (nonblanchable erythema), and 1 was Stage II (partial thickness). Overall incidence was 3.9% for the bunny boot, 4.6% for the egg crate, and 6.6% for the foot waffle (not significantly different among groups). The bunny boot with pillows was most cost effective (F[3], N = 240) = 1.342, p <= .001). CONCLUSIONS: In this study, the bunny boot was as effective as higher-tech devices. The results, however, were confounded by nurses adding pillows to the bunny boot group.
Journal Subset:	Core Nursing; Nursing; Peer Reviewed; USA

▮ FIGURE 2-2 Abbreviated Sample of a Full Citation Taken from *CINAHL* (http://www.ebscohost.com/cinahl/).

Research Resources

To simplify your search for evidence that can enhance your practice, it helps to be familiar with the major sources that publish research in nursing. Professional nursing journals are the most common resources for reports of research studies. There are two types of sources: nursing research journals and nursing clinical journals that contain a preponderance of research articles. Nursing research journals have as their primary focus the publication and dissemination of current research studies that are being conducted about relevant topics in nursing. The number of nursing research journals has grown significantly since the inception of the first journal *Nursing Research* in 1952. There are now nine mainstream nursing research journals, which we list and describe in Box 2-3. Note the range of articles available in the different journals.

Consider This . . .

How many of the journals in boxes 2-3 and 2-4 are you familiar with? How many have you read? You might want to check out several of the journals and sample the range of articles yourself.

BOX 2-3 Nursing Research Journals

Advances in Nursing Science—This quarterly journal features cutting edge research about the practice of nursing. Each issue is organized around a single research topic with implications for patient care. The format is unique in research journals as it does not adhere to the standard research report format. Recent 2010 topics have included:
- nursing essentials
- practice-based evidence

Applied Nursing Research—This quarterly journal features research that is directly tied to clinical applications across nursing specialties. A recent 2011 issue included:
- research articles on stroke awareness
- the management of foot ulcers in diabetics

Clinical Nursing Research—This quarterly journal features research that is directly tied to clinical nursing interventions. Recent 2011 issues included:
- research articles on oral care practices in the ICU
- mobility adaptations in older adults

Nursing Research—This is the original journal featuring research in nursing and it is published monthly. It covers a broad range of research studies across the spectrum of the profession of nursing. It also publishes articles about research and statistical methodologies. Sample 2011 articles included:
- patterns of anxiety in critically ill patients on mechanical ventilation
- effects of dietary fiber supplementation in individuals with fecal incontinence
- cluster analysis of intake, output, and voiding habits

Research in Nursing and Health—This bimonthly journal covers a wide range of research and theory including nursing practice, education, administration, nursing history, health issues, and research methods. Sample 2011 article topics included:
- testing whether modifications in bedrooms improved the sleep of new parents
- maternal role attainment with medically fragile infants

Research and Theory for Nursing Practice—This journal is published quarterly and covers theory and research for a wide range of nursing areas. Topics for 2011 articles included:
- comparing standards for determining adequate water intake for nursing home residents
- decision-making in caregivers of family members with heart failure

Southern Online Journal of Nursing Research—This online journal is published by the Southern Nursing Research Society and full text articles are available for free at http://snrs.org/publications/journal.html. Check out the site for sample articles.

continued . . .

continued . . .

Journal of Nursing Scholarship—This quarterly journal is published by Sigma Theta Tau Honor Society of Nursing and covers research focusing on the health of people worldwide. A sample of 2011 articles included:
- transnational mothers crossing the border and bringing their health care needs
- peer group intervention reduces personal HIV risk for Malawian health workers

Western Journal of Nursing Research—This journal is published eight times a year and covers nursing research from a broad and international perspective. It offers a unique feature with commentaries on the research studies and an author response to those commentaries. Sample 2008 articles included:
- a randomized controlled trial of breastfeeding support and education for adolescent mothers
- stress, coping, and well-being in military spouses during deployment separation

There are a large number of clinical specialty journals that also make research their focus. Usually at least half of their content is devoted to research studies in the specialty area covered by the journal. You can see a listing of just a few of these clinical journals in Box 2-4. Note the different specialties represented.

BOX 2-4 Sample Nursing Clinical Journals That Feature Research Studies

American Journal of Critical Care
AORN Journal
Cancer Nursing
Cardiovascular Nursing
Clinical Journal of Oncology Nursing
Critical Care Nursing Quarterly
Heart and Lung: Journal of Critical Care
Issues in Comprehensive Pediatric Nursing
Issues in Mental Health Nursing
Journal of Child and Adolescent Psychiatric Nursing
Journal of Community Health Nursing
Journal of Emergency Room Nursing
Journal of Obstetric, Gynecologic, and Neonatal Nursing
Journal of Pediatric Health Care
Journal of Pediatric Nursing: Nursing Care of Children and Families
Journal of Pediatric Oncology Nursing
Journal of Perinatal and Neonatal Nursing
Journal of School Nursing
Journal of the Society of Pediatric Nurses
MCN: The American Journal of Maternal/Child Nursing
Neonatal Network-Journal of Neonatal Nursing
Oncology Nursing Forum
Pediatric Nursing
Public Health Nursing
Rehabilitation Nursing

Other potentially useful journals that feature research studies include *Nursing Science Quarterly, Qualitative Health Research, Biological Research for Nursing, Journal of Nursing Education,* and *Nursing Administration Quarterly.*

There are also resources that feature reviews or summaries of nursing research. The most prominent of these is the *Annual Review of Nursing Research,* which selects a health care topic and collects all relevant nursing research on that topic for that year. It presents summaries and expert reviews of these articles in one volume. The 2010 volume had a focus on workforce issues.

Using articles that present integrated literature reviews can provide great resources for finding evidence-based information. We have already discussed the integrative literature reviews that can be found in the Cochrane databases. You will also find integrated reviews in the various research journals that we have identified. Another excellent resource for systematic reviews of research comes from the Agency for Healthcare Research and Quality (AHRQ). This agency produces periodic evidence reports on specified topics designed to improve the quality of health care offered in the United States. A complete listing of these reports can be found online at http://www.ahrq.gov /clinic/epcquick.htm.

You will also see newspaper or magazine articles that take information from healthcare research studies and report on research that might alert the general public to current and important issues in health care. See the "Research in the News" box below for an example.

Resource and Subject Matter

Research in the News

Handwashing: Does Your Doctor Do It Often Enough?

Point of View, CBC News, June 17, 2010

Doctors, nurses and other health-care professionals at several Vancouver Island hospitals aren't practising proper hygiene, according to an audit conducted into handwashing techniques.

Health professionals were openly observed for the entire month last February *at Victoria General, Royal Jubilee, Saanich Peninsula and Nanaimo General hospitals. The audit showed that less than one-third of all handwashing is done properly and that physicians are the worst offenders.*

On average, they were in compliance 12 per cent of the time.

The head of infection prevention and control for the heath authority, Bev Dobbin, called the results "surprising" and "disappointing."

Here is a news article on handwashing compliance.

What can you take from this article?

How might you go about locating the original audit information that this article was based on?

What does this tell you about how information from a research study reaches the general public?

SUMMARY

Finding evidence to support nursing practice depends on understanding and conducting effective searches. Here is a summary of the key points in this chapter.

- The ability to **search** and retrieve pertinent resources is key to finding evidence that supports the use of best nursing practices. Research studies and systematic reviews provide the best resources for obtaining current evidence. **Databases** and **bibliographic databases** provide lists of **citations** of published information about a topic, and may also include **abstracts** of the studies and reviews they cite. **Electronic databases** are computer accessible. *(Objective 1)*

- Successful retrieval of needed resources depends heavily on the selection of appropriate databases and the skillful use of search techniques. The *CINAHL* and **MEDLINE** databases are the two most comprehensive search tools for locating materials in nursing and health related disciplines. Some versions of these databases offer **full text** access to their articles, while others index thousands of **periodicals**. The **Cochrane Collaborative** offers CDSR and DARE, two useful database sets for locating **systematic reviews** about the usefulness of specific health care related interventions. *(Objective 2)*

- A search strategy is essential to make a search comprehensive and productive. Key steps in any search strategy include defining and focusing the topic for the search by setting **search limits** and using appropriate key words, selecting appropriate resources and databases, defining specific **search parameters** and **Boolean operators**, examining and using the search results, and collecting resources from the search. *(Objective 3)*

- Professional nursing journals are the best source for locating evidence-based resources. Nursing research journals focus on reporting current research studies. Clinical nursing journals report research that is pertinent to their clinical focus. *(Objective 4)*

STUDENT ACTIVITIES

Now it is time for you to see whether you can apply what you have learned.

1. Check out your academic library. Find out if they offer either online or face to face classes on using library resources such as databases and running searches. If these are available, take advantage of these services.

2. Explore the difference between an electronic database and a search engine. Are search engines ever appropriate when mounting a search for the best evidence for nursing practice?

3. Let's run an experiment. Try using a search engine to determine the best practices for handwashing. Use the key term handwashing. Now run the search in *CINAHL.* What differences do you see?

4. The following two articles examine strategies to increase compliance with hand-washing. One is a research article and one is a clinical narrative article. Locate and read both articles.

   a. Siegel, J.H. and D.M. Korniewicz. 2007. Keeping patients safe: an interventional hand hygiene study at an oncology center. *Clinical Journal of Oncology Nursing, 11(5)*: 643–646

   b. No authors. 2010. An ED makes changes to achieve compliance: some strategies worked better than others. *ED Nursing, 13(5)*: 55

Now that you have read both articles, what differences do you see? Which article has the best evidence of whether the identified practices were effective in increasing handwashing compliance?

Visit the web site and work the web exercises designed for this chapter.

Pearson Nursing Student Resources

Find additional review materials at
www.nursing.pearsonhighered.com
Prepare for success with additional NCLEX®-style practice questions, interactive assignments and activities, web links, animations and videos, and more!

REFERENCES

http://www.ebscohost.com/

CINAHL at http://www.ebscohost.com/cinahl/

Cochrane at http://www.cochrane.org/

Handwashing: Does your doctor do it often enough? (CBC News June 17, 2010) http://www.cbc.ca /news/pointofview/2010/06/handwashing-does -your-doctor-do-it-often-enough.html

http://academic.lexisnexis.com/

PubMed at http://www.ncbi.nlm.nih.gov/pubmed/

Stewart, S. and J.S. Box-Panksepp. 2004. Preventing hospital-acquired pressure ulcers: a point prevalence study. *Ostomy Wound Management*, *50*(3): 46–48, 50–51.

Makhsous, M., M. Priebe, J. Bankard, D. Rowles, M. Zeigler, D. Chen, and F. Lin. 2007. Measuring tissue perfusion during pressure relief maneuvers: insights into preventing pressure ulcers. *Journal of Spinal Cord Medicine*, *30*(5): 497–507.

CHAPTER

3

Research: A Process

CHAPTER OUTLINE

CHAPTER OBJECTIVES

1. Define the terms research, nursing research, and clinical nursing research.
2. Describe the five global phases of the research process.
3. Describe the circular nature of the research process.
4. Compare and contrast the research and nursing processes.

KEY TERMS

Clinical nursing research **(45)**

Deductive reasoning **(p. 46)**

Inductive reasoning **(p. 48)**

Nursing research **(p. 45)**

Research **(p. 45)**

Research process **(p. 46)**

Research proposal **(p. 47)**

ABSTRACT

Research is a process used to conduct systematic inquiries into identified problems and questions to find answers that generate or refine knowledge. Nursing research examines issues that are important to nursing in order to expand the foundations of nursing knowledge and expertise. Clinical nursing research provides answers to clinical problems that allow nurses to provide clinical care that is grounded on a solid scientific foundation.

This chapter is designed to give you a feel for what research is and to help you form a picture of research as a process. We will examine the concept of research and explore the phases of the research process. You will add some key research terminology to your vocabulary that will prove useful as we progress to the classification and application of research studies in the chapters to come.

Research: Introducing the Broad View

The newspaper headlines proclaimed "Nanotubes seen as new weapon in cancer fight" (Ackerman 2007). The story reviewed a study done by a team at MD Anderson Cancer Center that reported on a breakthrough technique which destroyed liver cancer tumors in rabbits with no side effects or damage to healthy cells. The research study was performed on rabbits in a controlled laboratory environment. The rabbits with liver cancer were given a treatment where the researchers injected carbon nanotubes into the rabbits' liver tumors and then exposed them to radio waves that heated the nanotubes and destroyed the cancer cells. These cells were then excreted from the body as waste. The treatment did no damage to any of the surrounding healthy tissues (Ackerman 2007).

This study fits perfectly with a predominant preconceived notion of what "research" is all about. You can almost picture a group of highly serious looking individuals in lab coats and safety goggles injecting dozens of rabbits with microscopic nanotubes and then strapping them to a table and beaming their precisely located livers with radio waves. We often picture research as something that happens in a brightly-lit chrome and steel laboratory setting far from day-to-day realities. However, whether you realize it or not, research and the results from research are an integral part of our lives. Billions of public and private dollars are spent each year on a wide array of research endeavors.

Consider This . . .

Stop for a minute and reflect on the world around you. What evidence of research do you see in your everyday life?

Research is used as a tool to evaluate and sell every type of product imaginable from drugs to toilet paper. Surveys are routinely conducted to provide information about what the public thinks or feels about a variety of subjects from politics to religion to some Hollywood actor's latest antics. Electronic "cookies" inhabit our computers and collect data on our Internet buying habits and then transmit that data back to some market research firm to analyze and interpret. Every time we shop and pay by credit card, someone is gathering information about what we bought in hopes of forecasting consumer trends. Companies survey our television viewing habits and analyze the data to make decisions about which shows stay on the air based on the data collected. All of these examples show research in action, as does the *Research in the News* box on page 43.

Research is blooming in the scientific community as well. Researchers continually develop new technologies for improving human life. For instance, the mapping of the human genome has led to an explosion of medical studies searching for etiologies of various diseases in hopes of eventually unlocking the key to a cure. Our example of using nanotube technology in combination with radio waves to kill cancer cells is amazing and may one day revolutionize the way we treat cancer. While not so well recognized, the nursing profession has also long been actively involved in conducting research. This research has made and continues to make important contributions to the health care arena.

You might make a case that the first nurse researcher was Florence Nightingale. She has been called a pioneer of the "notion that social phenomena could be objectively measured and subjected to mathematical analysis" (Cohen 1984, 128). She addressed many nursing issues in her day by identifying the problems, collecting and analyzing data, and proposing changes in care practices as a result of her studies. For example, she kept voluminous records of observations on sanitation and hygiene practices during the Crimean war. She subjected those records to extensive analysis and applied the results in the clinical area as well as writing her now well-known report entitled *Notes on Matters Affecting the Health, Efficiency and Hospital Administration . . .* (Nightingale 1858). This report led to the establishment of the British Royal Sanitary Commission.

Dumas and Leonard (1963) were the first nurses to conduct a true experimental research study in the clinical area when they investigated the effects of preoperative preparation in reducing vomiting in the immediate post-operative recovery period. They randomly assigned patients to a control and a treatment group. The treatment group got preoperative preparation while the control group did not. The frequency of post-operative vomiting was then measured postoperatively in both groups. The group that received preparation for surgery had less vomiting after surgery. Chapter 5 explores quantitative studies such as this in more detail, including an examination of specific experimental research designs.

Nurses have been instrumental in conducting enumerable research studies that have provided breakthroughs in the way health care is administered. Dr. Barbara Hansen (1979) was concerned that many of her patients experienced diarrhea when they were on a tube-fed diet. Research by Dr. Hansen and a consortium of colleagues eventually led to the use of a lactose-free dietary formula for tube feedings.

Research in the News

Really? The Claim: A Soap-and-Water Rinse Gets Produce Cleanest

BY ANAHAD O'CONNOR
The New York Times, October 4, 2010

THE FACTS The prospect of ingesting pesticides and other contaminants can make supermarket produce seem less than appetizing. Buying organic lowers the risk, but is no guarantee against food-borne pathogens.

Scientists have found some effective household measures that can eliminate germs and pesticides. The simplest? Rinsing with tap water, which works as well as a mild soap solution or fruit and vegetable washes.

In studies at the Connecticut Agricultural Experiment Station in 2000, for example, scientists compared pesticide removal methods on 196 samples of lettuce, strawberries and tomatoes. Some were rinsed under tap water for a minute; others were treated with either a 1 percent solution of Palmolive or a fruit and vegetable wash. Tap water "significantly reduced" residues of 9 of 12 pesticides, and it worked as well as soap and wash products, the studies found.

For micro-organisms, try rinsing produce with a mild solution of vinegar, about 10 percent. In a 2003 study at the University of Florida, researchers tested disinfectants on strawberries contaminated with E. coli and other germs. They found the vinegar mixture reduced bacteria by 90 percent and viruses by about 95 percent.

THE BOTTOM LINE To remove pesticides and germs, rinse produce with a vinegar solution, then wash with tap water for at least 30 seconds.

Here is a story in the *New York Times* that was drawn from two research studies.

- How might this article be useful in your everyday life?
- Does the fact that the information was taken from research studies make you feel any more confident about the advice being offered? Why or why not?

Check out one of the actual research studies at:

1. Krol, W.J., T.L. Arsenault, H.M. Pylypiw, M.J.I. Mattina. 2000. Reduction of Pesticide Residues on Produce by Rinsing. *Journal of Agriculture and Food Chemistry.* 48(10): 4666–4670.

2. Lukasik, J., M.L. Bradley, T.M. Scott, M. Dea, A. Koo, W.Y. Hsu, J.A. Bartz, and S.R. Farrah. 2003. Reduction of poliovirus 1, bacteriophages, Salmonella montevideo, and Escherichia coli O157:H7 on strawberries by physical and disinfectant washes. *Journal of Food Protection.* 66(2): 188–193.

Having read one of these studies carefully, do you feel that the *New York Times* writer accurately reported the results? If you were a reporter writing an article on the study for your local paper, what additional results would you have included, if any?

The popular FACES pain rating scale that is used to rate the level of pain in children was constructed beginning in 1981 by a pediatric nurse. She was working with young children who were burned and having difficulty communicating that pain. She observed misunderstandings between staff and the children and generally poor pain control. So Dr. Donna Wong and a colleague, Connie Baker, a child life specialist, decided that there needed to be a better method to assess pain in these children. They spent several years creating, revising, and testing what came to be known as the Wong-Baker FACES scale (Wong and Baker 1988). Dr. Molly Dougherty, a woman's health nurse practitioner, has done extensive work in identifying and treating urinary incontinence in older women. In 1985, she developed an intravaginal balloon device (IVBD) for measuring pelvic floor muscle contractions (Dougherty et al. 1986). This device has proved to be a valuable asset in determining whether an exercise regimen is effectively strengthening pelvic muscles and decreasing incontinence.

Consider This . . .

Can you think of a scientific discovery made by a nurse? Have you met a nurse researcher? If so, describe that experience and what it meant to you.

In each of these examples, nurses identified a need in clinical practice and conducted research that provided a solution. Nurses now routinely use these solutions in their practices. These examples are not isolated incidents. Nurses have long tackled and researched clinical problems to find viable solutions to those problems. A wonderful resource that presents a review of scientific breakthroughs in nursing from 1960 through 1999 has been compiled by Dr. Sue Donaldson (2000). You might want to peruse this review. It paints a vivid and broadly brushed picture of the recent evolution in nursing research. You will find the citation in the reference list at the end of this chapter.

Research Conceptualized

We touched briefly on the definition of research in Chapter 1. Now we are going to investigate the concept in more detail. In the broadest sense, research is a search for truth. Literally the term *research* means to "re- search" or to "search again".

A look at quickly accessible resources such as Wikipedia or the dictionary can be useful to form an initial impression. However, please keep in mind that while Wikipedia is a convenient source to begin to gather information, it lacks the reliability to serve as an authoritative source of information. Having set that boundary, *Wikipedia* defines research as a "human activity based on intellectual investigation and aimed at discovering, interpreting, and revising human knowledge on different aspects of the world" (http://en.wikipedia.org/wiki/Research). The *Merriam Webster Online Dictionary* defines research in part as a "studious inquiry or examination; *especially*: investigation or experimentation aimed at the discovery and interpretation of facts, revision of accepted theories or laws in the light of new facts, or practical application of such new or revised theories or laws" (www.webster.com/dictionary/research).

Now let's examine some more definitive resources. *Mosby's Dictionary of Medicine, Nursing & Health professions* (2008) defines research as the "diligent inquiry or examination of data, reports and observations in a search for facts or principles."

Resource and Subject Matter

One of the most widely recognized definitions of research is by Fred Kerlinger, a behavioral scientist. He described scientific research as a "systematic, controlled, empirical, and critical investigation of hypothetical propositions about the presumed relations among natural phenomena" (Kerlinger 1964, 11). This definition is densely packed with technical terms and is focused on experimental research. We will examine the different types of research and their characteristics in Chapters 5 and 6. A more easily understood definition was offered by Faye Abdellah. She was a pioneer in the field of nursing research and author of an early textbook on nursing research that defined research as "an activity whose purpose is to find a valid answer to some question that has been raised" (Abdellah and Levine 1965, 707).

A review of a number of current nursing research textbooks reveals remarkably similar definitions of the term "research." Polit and Beck (2011) define research as a "systematic inquiry that uses disciplined methods to answer questions or solve problems" (p. 3). They go on to state that "the ultimate goal of research is to develop, refine and expand a body of knowledge" (p. 3). Burns and Grove (2010) state that "research is a diligent systematic inquiry or study that validates and refines existing knowledge and develops new knowledge" (p. 4). Langford (2001) states that research "employs a systematic process to ask and answer questions that generate knowledge" (p. 74).

You will note that all of these definitions contain similar elements. We identify five critical elements of research:

1. It involves investigation and inquiry: This is a search that implies more than casual scrutiny.
2. It formulates questions or problems: Research is focused on relevant, useful, and important questions/problems. The question serves to bring focus and purpose to the investigation.
3. It is systematic: This emphasizes organization and planning and infers the use of a structured process.
4. It discovers answers: The goal of research is to find answers to the problems/questions raised.
5. It expands the knowledge base: The ultimate goal of research is to develop and refine knowledge.

Let's pull key elements from these definitions to form a more complete picture of the concept of research. **Research** is an investigation or inquiry of questions or problems which is conducted in a systematic manner to discover answers that expand the base of knowledge.

Now that we have defined research, the next question might be what is nursing research? Quite simply **nursing research** is research that focuses on questions or problems that are important to the profession of nursing. This includes questions raised in nursing practice, nursing education, and nursing administration. Issues that confront the nursing profession itself can also be researched. Nurses use research as a tool to produce and refine their knowledge. In this textbook, we will focus on **clinical nursing research**, which addresses problems in a clinical setting. It is designed to provide answers that will better guide nursing practice to improve the health status and care of individuals who require nursing services. Some examples of clinical nursing research studies can be seen in Box 3-1. As you can see, the issues nursing research investigates are highly relevant to the everyday practice of nursing.

BOX 3-1 Examples of Clinical Nursing Research Studies

Example 1
A study was conducted to test whether cardiac index measurements for normothermic patients were any different when room temperature injectates versus iced injectates were used. [Walsh, E., et al. (2010). Iced vs room-temperature injectates for cardiac index measurement during hypothermia and normothermia. *American Journal of Critical Care, 19*(4): 365–372.]

Example 2
A study was conducted to compare temporal artery and rectal temperature measurements in children. [Carr, E., et al. (2011). Comparison of temporal artery to rectal temperature measurements in children up to 24 months. *Journal of Pediatric Nursing, 26*(3): 179–185.]

Example 3
A pilot study was conducted to test the effectiveness of a protocol designed to increase breastfeeding in first time mothers. [McQueen, K., Dennis, C., Stremler, R., and Norman, C. (2011). A Pilot randomized controlled trial of a breastfeeding self-efficacy intervention with primiparous mothers. *Journal of Obstetric, Gynecologic, & Neonatal Nursing, 40*(1): 35–46.]

Example 4
A study was conducted to determine whether use of abdominal massage in addition to laxatives was effective for people with chronic constipation. [Lamas, K., Lindholm, L., Engstrom, B., and Jacobsson, C. (2010). Abdominal massage for people with constipation: a cost utility analysis. *Journal of Advanced Nursing, 66*(8): 1719–1729.]

Research Process

The **research process** is a circular process that contains a series of phases and steps. These phases move us from asking a question to finding an answer and then using that answer in practice. The answers that we find sow the seeds for new questions and this starts the process again. Figure 3-1 illustrates the phases and the cyclical nature of the process. Each phase of this research process builds on the one before it, deepening the researcher's understanding of the problem to be addressed. We will build upon this figure in Chapters 4, 5, and 7 as we fill in the steps that are used for each phase.

Phase 1: Conceptualize the Problem

In this phase of the research process, the researcher tries to determine what to study. The thought process uses **deductive reasoning** as the researcher starts with a general area of interest and breaks it down to more specific parts. This interest may arise from a situation in the clinical area where there is some recognition of an issue or difficulty or of a problem that exists. Perhaps the researcher has a certain theory that he/she wishes to examine and test. During this phase, the researcher thinks, reflects, reads, and confers with colleagues about the idea. Decisions are made here about what to study and what not to study as well as who to study. The researcher is trying to make decisions about how to frame and focus the study.

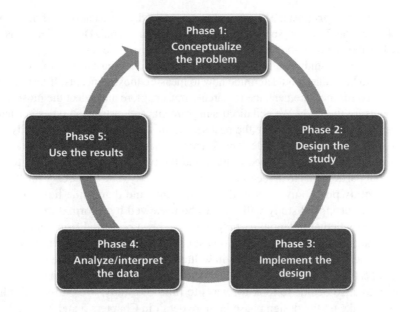

FIGURE 3-1 The Research Process
The five phases of research guide this circular process.

The researcher also needs to place the idea into some kind of context. As we saw in Chapter 2, literature searches help to determine how a line of inquiry fits into what has already been studied. The idea must be clarified, refined, and hammered into a useable problem or question. The idea must be researchable, meaning that it must address a problem that can be directly or indirectly observed. Research does not deal with philosophical or moral issues such as whether the use of stem cells is right or whether abortion is a moral choice. The focus of the study must be relevant and important to the practice of nursing. The study must also be feasible. This involves assessing whether there are sufficient resources (time, money, facilities, personnel) and expertise to carry out the proposed research study. As Chapter 4 discusses, these practical issues must be addressed to ensure a successful study.

Consider This . . .

Can you think of some ideas in nursing that might need researching? Hint: Think of a clinical skill that you have learned recently. Ask yourself: "How effective is . . .?"

This phase is largely an intellectual exercise as options and directions are considered, then discarded or revised and refined. This phase calls for creative thought and insight. It cannot be rushed through as it forms the foundation for the rest of the study. The final conceptualization of the problem must be firmly grounded in the literature and be sufficiently refined to provide a feasible foundation for study. Once this occurs the researcher moves to Phase 2.

Phase 2: Design the Study

In this phase the researcher makes plans about how the study will be carried out. A study is ultimately only as good as its design. This phase involves drawing up a formal plan known as a **research proposal**. The researcher must first decide what type of design to use. Chapters 4, 5, 6, and 7 discuss specific design types in more detail. Design decisions are often dictated by the nature of the problem and the philosophy of the researcher, and the design in turn affects how the study will be carried out. The researcher must also define the concepts that are going to be studied and determine how to measure those concepts. If instruments are going to be used for measurement, the researcher must explore and select the most appropriate instruments for the study. We will discuss instruments and instrument types in Chapter 5.

The researcher must determine the best setting in which to conduct the study and determine if such a setting is available. The researcher needs to decide what characteristics the potential study participants need to have and the best ways to gain access to and get these potential participants to agree to be a part of the study. The researcher must consider whether the study poses any risks to the participants and determine how to minimize those risks. The proposed study will have to be reviewed by a formal review committee to determine whether potential participants have been protected from harm. Once the various decisions are made about how to best conduct the study, a research proposal is drawn up that details all of the decisions in written form. At this point the researcher may have the plan critiqued by peers or consultants to get feedback on the plan's viability. The researcher may also decide to look for ways to fund the study. We will revisit all these elements that make up the design phase in more detail in Chapters 5 and 7.

Phase 3: Implement the Design

This phase is fairly straightforward and involves activating the plans laid out in Phase 2 by collecting the data that is needed. This can be an exciting time in the process as the researcher sees the plan in action and senses that the study will be completed. However, this phase also presents challenges as studies are seldom conducted without some hitch or glitch in the process. These hitches mean that the researcher needs to be intimately involved and fully informed as the process of collecting data proceeds. Study implementation is often a time that calls for quick thinking and creative problem solving to adapt the plan as needed to ensure the collection of useable and credible data. I can now look back with humor at some of the problems that have occurred to me or my colleagues during the collection of data. However, at the time, they seemed like disasters of major proportion. Perhaps one of the most memorable was when the clinic that we were using as a data collection site declared bankruptcy and promptly closed down. We were fortunate enough to locate another clinic and carry on.

Phase 4: Analyze/Interpret the Data

In this phase, the researcher focuses on analyzing and interpreting the data that was collected in Phase 3. Data in its raw form is not particularly useful to the consumer of research. The researcher must use methods to translate those raw bits of data into some kind of meaningful and useful picture. This means coming up with definitive answers to the problems or questions that were posed back in Phase 1 of the process. Statistics are frequently used to succinctly describe the data and seek these answers, as we will see in Chapter 5. It also means interpreting the results so that we know what those answers mean and how they are relevant to the practice of nursing. Here the researcher uses an **inductive reasoning** process (moving from the specific to the general) as the specific results of the study are compared to the literature and placed in a larger nursing context. The results are also examined to see whether they might be used in clinical practice, and if so in what manner.

Phase 5: Use the Results

Knowledge gained is never final; it always plants seeds that bear the fruit of ongoing investigation. In other words, the answers and the application of those answers start to generate new questions and new problems, making research a cyclical process. It is the researcher's job to make recommendations for further research in this phase. The final job of the researcher is to disseminate the results so that they may be read by other nurses and health care providers. At this point, it is the job of the research consumer (you) to read and apply these results in pursuit of professional practice. The use of research-generated knowledge is a part of the practicing nurse's obligation to keep his/her nursing practices current and grounded on a solid scientific base.

Chapters 5 and 7 explore these phases in greater depth and examine the specific steps that fall under each phase. You will see that the phases are applied somewhat differently depending on whether the researchers are conducting quantitative or qualitative research.

Comparing the Research Process to the Nursing Process

Research as a process may seem familiar to you because it is a lot like the nursing process. Both processes involve a purpose, a series of actions, and a goal. They both require critical thinking and problem solving abilities. There are a number of similarities in the two processes. They are both divided into five phases. They both involve identifying and refining a problem, planning to address the problem, implementing the plan, and analyzing the results of any actions taken. You can compare the two processes in Table 3-1.

▶ Table 3-1   Comparing the Nursing and Research Processes

Nursing Process	Research Process
Assessment (determine what is going on, and what it means)	**Conceptualize the problem** (identify felt need, review the literature)
Diagnosis (name the problem)	**Conceptualize the problem** (define problem, identify purpose, describe scope)
Planning (identify actions to alleviate the problem)	**Design the study** (determine who is studied, how to study them, and how to measure the concepts being studied)
Implementation (put the plan into action)	**Implement the design** (collect the data)
Evaluation (determine if actions were effective and resolved the problem; if not, determine modifications that need to be made in the plan)	**Analyze/interpret the data** (answer the research questions) **Use the Results** (apply results to nursing practice)

You will discover as we continue our journey together that the research process is more complex than the nursing process. Each of the phases in the research process contain a number of sub-steps, and these steps and their order may differ by the type of study that is proposed. Research also has a specialized language and vocabulary that must be interpreted, as well as a variety of specialized methods, designs, and possible approaches. You will learn the vocabulary that is necessary to understand the research process as you progress through this book.

Consider This . . .

In what ways does comparing the research process to the nursing process enhance your general understanding of what the research process is? What differences do you see in the two processes?

The theoretical foundations needed to put the research process in motion are more substantial than the theory that undergirds the nursing process. All the phases of the research process are logically linked to one another and grounded in theory that forms the base for the study. Conducting a research study requires greater accuracy, thoroughness, and direction than implementing the nursing process. While the nursing process is narrowly focused on the clinical arena, the research process can focus on clinical, educational, and/or professional arenas. Research outcomes have much broader implications for practice and are shared with a much wider audience while the nursing process focuses on the patient and family. The research process leads to research outcomes that are often used to alter nursing practices while the nursing process guides the use of the best practices available in a specified situation.

SUMMARY

In this chapter, you have examined definitions for research, nursing research, and clinical nursing research. You have been introduced to the research process and its five attendant phases. Finally, we have compared the research process to the nursing process. Here is a summary of the key points in this chapter.

- Florence Nightingale was the first nurse researcher and pioneered the use of empirical knowledge to improve nursing practice. **Research** is defined as an investigation or inquiry of questions or problems which is conducted in a systematic manner to discover answers that expand the base of knowledge. **Nursing research** is research that focuses on questions or problems that are important to the profession of nursing and includes questions raised in nursing practice, nursing education, and nursing administration. **Clinical nursing research** is research that is designed to provide answers to specifically identified clinical problems in order to better guide nurses in the administration of patient care. *(Objective 1)*

- The **research process** is comprised of five broad phases: Phase 1 of the process is a conceptual exercise in which the researcher uses **deductive reasoning** to produce a clearly defined and feasible research problem that is grounded in the literature. In Phase 2, the researcher selects a design and presents plans for how to carry out the study in a **research proposal.** Phase 3 is the implementation phase, in which the researcher activates the research plan and collects data. In Phase 4, the researcher uses **inductive reasoning** to analyze and interpret the date that was collected in Phase 3. Phase 5 focuses on how to share and use the results of the study and makes recommendations for future research. *(Objective 2)*

- The five phases and steps of the research process form a circular process. This circular process moves us from asking a question to finding an answer and then using that answer in practice. The answers that we find then sow the seeds for new questions and the circle is complete and the process starts again. *(Objective 3)*

- The nursing process and research process share many similar characteristics. They both involve a purpose, a plan, a series of actions, a goal, analysis and evaluation, and require critical thought. However, the research process is more global in scope and is ultimately more complex than the nursing process. Outcomes from the research process provide evidence for and dictate the best practices for nursing. *(Objective 4)*

STUDENT ACTIVITIES

Now it is time for you to see whether you can apply what you have learned.

1. View this YouTube video on *Nurse Scientists* at www.youtube.com/watch?v =8YIAB1nOfro&feature=related. What did you discover about nursing research? How did it make you feel about choosing nursing as a profession?

2. Why is it important for us as nurses to understand the research process even if we never conduct a research study?

3. What changes do you see happening in health care that need to be researched?

4. Run a search on the web for definitions of the term "research". What are the common elements in the definitions you discovered? Would you add anything to the critical elements that were identified on page 45 in this chapter?

Resource and Subject Matter

Pearson Nursing Student Resources

Find additional review materials at

www.nursing.pearsonhighered.com

Prepare for success with additional NCLEX®-style practice questions, interactive assignments and activities, web links, animations and videos, and more!

REFERENCES

Abdellah, F.G. and E. Levine. 1965. *Better patient care through nursing research*. New York, NY: Macmillan.

Ackerman, T. 2007. Nanotubes seen as new weapon in cancer fight. *Houston Chronicle*. pp. A1, A5.

Burns, N. and S.K. Grove. 2010. *Understanding Nursing Research, building an evidence-based practice*. (5th ed.) St. Louis, MO: Saunders.

Carr, E., M. Wilmoth, A. Eliades, J. Baker, D. Shelestak, K. Heisroth, and K. Stoner. 2011. Comparison of temporal artery to rectal temperature measurements in children up to 24 months. *Journal of Pediatric Nursing, 26*(3): 179–185.

Cohen, I.B. 1984. Florence Nightingale. *Scientific American, 250*(3): 128–137.

Donaldson S. 2000. Breakthroughs in scientific research: The discipline of nursing, 1960-1999. *Annual Review of Nursing Research, 18,* 247–311.

Dougherty, M., R. Abrams, and L. McKey. 1986. An instrument to assess dynamic characteristics of circumvaginal musculature. *Nursing Research, 35*(4): 202–206.

Dumas, R.G. & R.C. Leonard. 1963. The effect of nursing on the incidence of post operative vomiting. *Nursing Research, 12*(1): 12–15.

Hansen, B.C., N. Bergstrom, M. Grant, R. Hanson, M. Heitkemper, W. Kubo, et al. 1979. Nursing interventions in problems of tube feeding, a consortium project. *American Nurses Association Publications,* (D-67): 8–9.

Kerlinger, F.N. 1964. *Foundations of behavioral research.* Austin, TX: Holt, Rinehart and Winston.

Lamas, K., L. Lindholm, B. Engstrom, and C. Jacobsson. 2010. Abdominal massage for people with constipation: a cost utility analysis. *Journal of Advanced Nursing, 66*(8): 1719–1729.

Langford, R.W. 2001. *Navigating the maze of nursing research.* St. Louis, MO: Mosby.

McQueen, K., C. Dennis, R. Stremler, and C. Norman. 2011. A pilot randomized controlled trial of a breastfeeding self-efficacy intervention with primiparous mothers. *Journal of Obstetric, Gynecologic, & Neonatal Nursing, 40*(1): 35–46.

Merriam-Webster Online Dictionary at http://www.webster.com/dictionary/research

Mosby's Dictionary of medicine, nursing & health professions 2008 (8th ed) St Louis, MO: Mosby at Elsevier.

Nightingale, F. 1858. *Notes on matters affecting the health, efficiency and hospital administration of the British army founded chiefly on the experience of the late wars.* London, UK: Harrison and Sons.

Polit, D.F. and C.T. Beck. 2011. *Nursing research, generating and assessing evidence for nursing practice.* (9th ed.) New York, NY: Lippincott Williams & Wilkins.

Walsh, E., S. Adams, J. Chernipeski, J. Cloud, and E. Gillies. 2010. Iced vs room-temperature injectates for cardiac index measurement during hypothermia and normothermia. *American Journal of Critical Care, 19*(4): 365–372.

Wikipedia at http://en.wikipedia.org/wiki/Research

Wong, D. and C. Baker. 1988. Pain in children: comparison of assessment scales. *Pediatric Nursing, 14*(1): 9–17.

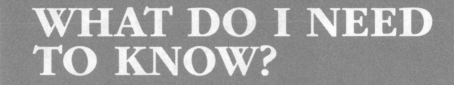

PART

II

WHAT DO I NEED TO KNOW?

. . . exploring quantitative and qualitative perspectives

learning the language, dissecting the process

Health care and health care delivery is expanding in geo-metric proportions and has become increasingly complex. The foundations for the practice of nursing are ever evolving. How do we keep our foundation solid and our practice current? Research is the key. It provides us tested information about the best practices in nursing. To effectively use this information, we need to understand the language of research. This section defines research, and introduces you to key terms that you will need in order to understand what you are reading when you peruse a research article. It explores both quantitative and qualitative research methodologies in detail and provides you with specific examples from actual nursing research studies.

Two Broad Research Traditions

CHAPTER OUTLINE

CHAPTER OBJECTIVES

1. Describe the philosophical origins of quantitative and qualitative research.
2. Compare and contrast quantitative and qualitative research methods.
3. Trace the evolution of ethical considerations to protect human subjects.
4. Explain the importance of ethical considerations in nursing research.

KEY TERMS

Anonymity (p. 72)

Assent (p. 70)

Belmont Report
 (p. 68)

Beneficence (p. 69)

Benefit (p. 69)

Confidentiality (p. 70)

Constructivism (p. 57)

Generalizable (p. 59)

Informed Consent (p. 70)

Institutional Review Board
 (IRB) (p. 70)

Justice (p. 69)

Phenomenon (p. 56)

Positivism (p. 56)

Quantitative Research
 (p. 56)

Qualitative Research (p. 57)

Respect for Persons (p. 69)

Risk (p. 69)

Scientific Misconduct (p. 72)

ABSTRACT

How research studies are developed is a process embedded in beliefs that investigators have about the development of scientific knowledge. Two very different approaches guide research development. Quantitative research grew out of a positivist tradition while qualitative research originated from a constructivist perspective. Traditionally, investigators use quantitative research techniques for the purposes of scientific discovery. While quantitative research has provided much valuable information, it does not tell the whole story about the practice of nursing. Many facets of nursing do not lend themselves to the highly structured methods of quantitative research. Thus, qualitative research that relies on less structured, narrative methods has made valuable contributions to the science of nursing. All research, whether quantitative or qualitative must consider the rights of the participants in the study.

This chapter explores philosophical perspectives underlying research methods, the commonalities and differences between quantitative and qualitative research, and the value of each of these modes of scientific discovery. The chapter also examines the history and processes associated with safeguarding the rights of research participants.

Philosophical Origins of Quantitative and Qualitative Research

Two broad methods of inquiry, quantitative and qualitative research, drive the systematic investigation of phenomena in health care. Derived from two different philosophical perspectives or paradigms, each method has a common goal of scientifically discovering new knowledge. However, each method approaches the process of discovery quite differently.

The specific aims of quantitative and qualitative research have different philosophical underpinnings. While both forms of research seek to discover the truth about how phenomena occur, each arises from a different philosophical position that influences the way researchers look at the world. Table 4-1 highlights key differences between the two philosophical views discussed in this section.

▶ Table 4-1   Differences in Philosophical Underpinnings of Research

	Positivist	Constructivist
Reality	Single reality: phenomena work in only one way which needs to be discovered	Multiple realities: how phenomena work depends on experiences and perspectives of individuals involved
Truth	Discovered through conduct of highly controlled studies that investigator designs based on current knowledge of the phenomenon	Relative to how people view world—to discover the view, investigators must ask people who know about the phenomenon
Goal	To explain, predict, and control phenomena	To discover how people make sense of world

Before getting started, a question one might ask is "what differences do philosophical perspectives or positions make in research?" In Chapter 3 research was conceptualized as a process composed of five phases. Figure 3-1 diagramed the connection of these phases. Philosophical positions provide the underpinnings for the research process. Imagine the research phases immersed in thinking that influences how individuals perceive science and the best approaches to study research problems. The pale blue background in Figure 4-1 represents the philosophical surroundings of science. The arrows indicate that the entire research process is embedded in and influenced by the underlying philosophical beliefs about the process of discovery. Two major philosophical positions that influence thinking about research are discussed.

Positivist Tradition

Philosophically, quantitative research has its roots in positivism. According to the tenets of **positivism**, scientists believe that a reality exists and that it can be discovered (Guba and Lincoln 1994). A single reality implies there is one truth that needs uncovered about a particular phenomenon. A **phenomenon** is an event that can be observed through the senses. Although positivists may not know exactly what the truth is, investigators believe it exists and systematically seek to discover it. Positivists believe that highly controlled experiments offer insight into reality. The purpose of positivist research is to explain, predict, and control phenomena (Guba and Lincoln 1994). In other words, scientists want to understand phenomena thoroughly in order to explain phenomena, predict what will happen if particular events occur, and control outcomes. Discovery occurs piece by piece or study by study. In this scheme, investigators use quantitative research to study a narrow and specific problem to see if insight into how a phenomenon works can be gleaned from the study outcome. **Quantitative research** systematically collects and analyzes numerical information. Each piece of new evidence gives insight into the truth about how reality functions. Multiple studies conducted over time test the theory and help to add to the body of evidence about a specific phenomenon. As a long-standing hallmark

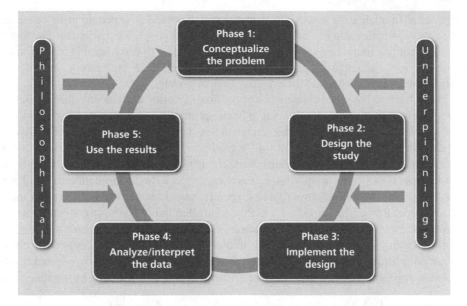

◼ FIGURE 4-1 Philosophical Position Surrounds and Influences Research Activities

Research is embedded in assumptions and beliefs. Philosophical underpinnings influence everything the investigator does.

of scientific discovery, the positivist perspective guided scientific exploration for several hundred years.

As an example, nursing has a scientific knowledge base regarding health promotion habits as a way to increase activity and decrease obesity. Getting people to participate routinely in health promotion activities is difficult. A positivist paradigm would be quite useful in guiding research to test a specific intervention for increasing health promotion participation in pregnant women. In other words, researchers are taking the theory that we have and designing a study to test that theory. Investigators would narrow the scope of study to a defined aspect of health promotion, design a structured intervention, and test that intervention to ascertain its effectiveness. Increased participation in health promotion activities as a result of the intervention would add support to the body of knowledge regarding engagement in health promotion. If the intervention were unsuccessful, investigators would return the drawing board trying to understand why the planned activities did not work. Based on these outcomes, investigators may modify their perspective about increasing health promotion participation and propose the next study.

Constructivist Tradition

While positivism has heavily influenced much quantitative research, its prescribed methods of discovery do not always capture the everyday realities of people's lives. Qualitative research adopts a somewhat different philosophical stance derived from constructivist thinking. Rather than positivist thinking that only one truth exists about how the world works, **constructivism** posits the stance that truth is relative to how people view the world (Guba and Lincoln 1994). Because people generate truth from their knowledge and experience, multiple perspectives can simultaneously exist. **Qualitative research** systematically gathers and analyzes narrative information. In qualitative research, the goal is to understand how people make sense out of their world—to develop an understanding derived from people's experiences. The highly controlled studies found in quantitative research are unable to discover this type of information. However, talking with people about their experiences in exploratory, unstructured situations offers new insight into the everyday lives of people.

Think back to the research example of health promotion activities. While we have a knowledge base regarding participation in health promoting activities, we also know that many people elect not to participate even when they recognize the value of the activities. Quantitative research studies cannot fully explain the many factors associated with participation in health promoting activities. Because insufficient information is known about specific aspects of health promotion, researchers explore the phenomenon to build new theory. Research from a constructivist perspective would study the issue from a much broader scope. Rather than structure a highly controlled intervention, investigators would begin to ask people about their participation in health promotion activities and the reasons for electing to engage or not engage in these behaviors. Researchers add the newly discovered information to the theoretical knowledge base and perspectives about health promotion shift. Investigators then determine the next steps for further investigation.

Importance of Philosophical Origins to Nursing Research

Why do basic philosophical perspectives make a difference in nursing research? Philosophical perspectives form the lens through which nurses perceive situations. Nursing practice takes place in clinical settings. The interventions nurses use have an impact on patients and families. From a positivist perspective, nurses want to know that these interventions are based on scientific evidence that explains what is happening and predicts outcomes of specific care measures. Controlled research helps to derive definitive answers to patient care problems. Yet patients and families are human beings who bring their personal life history to patient care situations. They and their health care providers bring many perspectives about the meaning of illness and have many expectations about health care. It is difficult to sort through the complexity of health care interactions and effectively intervene. A constructivist perspective acknowledges the multiplicity of views. Research from a constructivist perspective recognizes the diversity of perspectives and seeks to understand numerous outlooks that inform patient care situations.

> **Consider This . . .**
>
> Which perspective, positivist or constructivist, is better? What value might each perspective bring to the practice of nursing?

Quantitative and Qualitative Approaches

Both quantitative and qualitative research seek to gather and analyze information. However, qualitative research focuses on the gathering and analysis of narrative information. In the simplest terms, quantitative research employs numbers while qualitative research uses words. The scope of quantitative studies tends to be smaller because there is greater need to control the elements of the study. Control allows the researcher to manage factors outside of the study scope that might influence the outcomes. While the scope of the study is narrower, the number of subjects in quantitative research samples tends to be larger. Maximizing control over the research environment is the key to ensuring that conclusions derived from the study are generalizable to other similar groups. When study findings are **generalizable**, the findings of one study extend to other groups beyond those people participating in the study.

On the other hand, qualitative research gathers in-depth information about a phenomenon in natural settings with few controls. The detailed description resulting from qualitative research may uncover aspects of information not previously considered. The method allows for a broader scope of inquiry and gathering a greater depth of information. Because the information gathered has substantially greater depth than quantitative research, sample sizes tend to be smaller. The trade-off for this in-depth information is that generalizability of study findings to other groups is limited. Each method produces research findings that can be used in different ways. Both methods are valuable assets which add to the science base for nursing. Table 4-2 highlights some of the differences between quantitative and qualitative research.

To understand further the differences between quantitative and qualitative research, Boxes 4-1 and 4-2 present summaries of two articles. Box 4-1 summarizes a quantitative study about a cognitive behavioral intervention for women with Multiple Sclerosis (MS). Box 4-2 summarizes a qualitative study regarding experiences of individuals diagnosed with MS. Let's explore these studies in light of the key features of quantitative and qualitative research identified in Table 4-2.

Modes of Reasoning

Researchers apply one of two types of logic or reasoning to the research process. Quantitative research relies on deductive reasoning, in which thinking moves from general to specific, to set up experiments that test hypotheses about how phenomena work. In quantitative studies, researchers begin with a theoretical basis or premise and then apply it to a specific situation. Note how Sinclair and Scroggie's quantitative study (2005) followed the Lazarus and Folkman Stress and Coping Model, which suggests that stress is mediated by primary appraisal in which the strength of the stressor is assessed and followed by a secondary appraisal examining resources to meet the stressor. Information gained through these two appraisals influences the physical and psychological outcomes. This model spells out the general premises, which researchers applied to a specific research situation. They deduced or reasoned that an intervention influencing how individuals could cope with a diagnosis of MS would also influence the appraisals, thus reducing psychological and physical stress. Their article demonstrates the use of deduction in research. Researchers begin with the broad theoretical constructs and then tie them down to a specific research situation.

Inductive reasoning demonstrates the opposite process from deduction. Inductive reasoning applies information from a specific situation to a larger picture. Qualitative research relies on inductive thinking processes to explore the breadth and depth of a phenomenon. Researchers begin with a specific situation and from it derive a more general explanation. In the Barker-Collo et al. (2006) qualitative study on living with MS, researchers examined the experiences of 16 participants diagnosed with MS. In their summary statements, researchers broadened the application by highlighting the confusing nature of MS and the prevalence of discrimination and stigmatization associated with the disease. In this study researchers used inductive thinking beginning with the participants' individual situations, then expanded those experiences to a broader explanation of the impact of an MS diagnosis on the lives of people who receive it.

▶ Table 4-2 Key Differences between Quantitative and Qualitative Research

	Quantitative Research	Qualitative Research
Predominant Mode of Reasoning	Deductive	Inductive
Research Process	Highly structured	Fluid, flexible, iterative
Scope	Focuses on smaller number of specific concepts. Usually has larger sample sizes.	Attempts to understand the entirety of a phenomenon. Smaller samples sizes usually acceptable.
Preconceptions	Researchers base research questions or hypotheses on preconceived ideas of how study concepts interrelate. These facilitate development of research questions or hypotheses.	Researchers approach studies without preconceived ideas regarding study outcome. Method stresses importance of participants' interpretation of events and circumstances, rather than the researchers' ideas of what the research will "prove".
Setting/Conditions	Collects information under conditions of high control. For example: laboratories or use of structured study procedures.	Doesn't attempt to control the context of the research, but attempts to capture the picture in its entirety. For example: naturalistic settings.
Methods/ Instruments	Uses structured process and formal instruments for data collection.	Uses methods such as observation and interviewing for data collection. Researcher serves as instrument.
Analysis	Statistical analysis of numerical data. Researcher interprets statistical findings.	Logical analysis of narrative information. Analysis and data collection move back and forth. Researcher interprets narrative findings.

BOX 4-1 Summary of Quantitative Study

Sinclair, V. and J. Scroggie. 2005. Effects of a cognitive-behavioral program for women with multiple sclerosis. *Journal of Neuroscience Nursing, 37*(5): 249–257, 276.

Sinclair and Scroggie were two nurse researchers who wanted to design an intervention that would help women with multiple sclerosis (MS) cope more effectively with their disease.

Conceptual Framework
Using Lazarus and Folkman's Stress and Coping Model, researchers predicted that an intervention would increase the participants' sense of control over their MS. **[Preconception]** According to the theory, people's perceptions play an important role in how they adapt to stress. Beliefs about the strength of the stressor and about the ability to meet the challenge influence the coping behaviors that lead to psychological and physical outcomes.

Hypotheses
Researchers developed two hypotheses (a) "compared to preintervention scores, post intervention scores will reflect a positive impact on patients' perceptions of competence, coping behaviors, psychological well-being, and health related quality of life, and fatigue"; and (b) "compared to initial postintervention scores, 6-month follow-up scores indicating perceived health competence, coping behaviors, psychological well-being, health-related quality of life, and fatigue will reflect stabilization or improvement" (p. 251). **[Preconception]**

Sample
The final sample consisted of two groups totaling 37 women. **[Scope]** All women received the intervention. To control for potentially confounding variables, participants were female, had relapsing-remitting MS, and had a score of less than 6 on a disability status scale. **[Setting/ Condition]**

Intervention
The intervention was called a cognitive behavior program. The program consisted of five group sessions and a manual containing readings and exercises to promote use of the information covered in the group sessions. Sessions addressed (a) the mind-body connection; (b) role of unrealistic expectations in raising stress; (c) managing fears; (d) methods for managing anger and depression; and (e) enhancing social support through communication.

Measurement
Quantitative data were collected at four points in time during the study. **[Process]** The first measure was taken 5 weeks before the program began while the second measure was taken during the week before the program began. These two measures were considered baseline information because they were recorded prior to the intervention. The third measure was taken immediately after completing the program while the final measure was taken 6 months after program completion.

Several different instruments were used to collect data. **[Methods/Instruments]** During the first time measure, demographic data related to features such as age, education, marital status, race, and employment were collected. For all four measures researchers had participants fill out quantitative instruments that related to psychological and physical outcomes including those on personal coping resources, coping behavior, physical well-being, psychological well-being, and quality of life.

continued . . .

continued . . .

Analysis

Quantitative analyses were completed to statistically test the two hypotheses. Two statistical procedures—either a *t*-test or a Multiple Analysis of Variance (MANOVA) compared the different measures of the instruments. **[Analysis]**

Findings

The first hypothesis stating that participants would show significant improvements between their initial scores and post intervention was supported. Participants had significantly higher scores in their perceived competence, coping, psychological well-being, and quality of life. One area in which there was not significant improvement was related to physical outcomes.

The second hypothesis comparing the first post intervention scores to the 6-month follow-up scores on each of the instruments indicated that scores either stabilized or improved. This outcome means that even though the support groups had ended, the gains made during the intervention were present after the intervention or continued to improve 6 months following the intervention.

BOX 4-2 Summary of Qualitative Study

Barker-Collo, S., C. Cartwright, and J. Read. 2006. Into the unknown: The experiences of individuals living with multiple sclerosis. *Journal of Neuroscience Nursing, 38*(6): 435–441, 446.

Barker-Collo, Cartwright, and Reed wanted to better understand the experiences of individuals who had been diagnosed and were living with multiple sclerosis (MS).

Purpose

"The purpose of this study was to explore participants' prediagnostic and diagnostic experiences as well as the implications for living with the disease" (p. 436). **[Scope]**

Sample

Sixteen participants with a primary diagnosis of MS were recruited. Half of the participants had relapsing-remitting MS (RRMS) while the other half had primary progressive MS (PPMS). **[Scope]**

Procedures

Individual interviews using a semi-structured interview schedule **[Methods/Instruments]** were conducted in participant homes. **[Setting]** Interviews lasted from 1 to 2 hours and were audiotape recorded. Following the interview, tapes were transcribed verbatim.

Analysis

Each of the researchers independently reviewed the transcripts to familiarize themselves with the interviews. During subsequent review related data were grouped together and descriptively labeled according to the category. **[Analysis]**

Findings

The first themes that emerged were related to diagnosis of MS. The phases included the *Prediagnostic Stage* which reflected a growing awareness of what initially seemed like unrelated or transient symptoms that were minimized or ignored. During the *Diagnostic Experience* participants indicated a sense of powerlessness during the process. They felt helpless and experienced anxiety and fear. Even after diagnosis participants still felt powerless and described the initial moments of diagnosis with "trauma, shock, fear, anger and sometimes relief" (p. 437). In the theme *Reactions to Diagnosis* some participants indicated diagnosis sometimes was perceived as a relief because the disease was not cancer. However, participants felt scared and were also concerned for their family members.

The theme *Living with MS* reflected the impact that MS had on participant lives. Type of MS diagnosis made a difference. Those with RRMS shared about the variability of their disease and the uncertainty they faced from day to day. Those with PPMS expressed hopelessness and fear with regard to their eventual decline. On a positive note, many participants had made healthy lifestyle changes.

Research Process

Quantitative studies follow a highly structured research process. Researchers make an effort to systematically select study participants who are similar to a larger group of individuals who would benefit from application of study findings. Subjects may be assigned using a random process to treatment or regular care groups to ensure that the groups are similar in nature before the study begins. A clear set of instructions (protocol) guides uniform treatment of study participants and ensures consistent measurement methods. In the study of a cognitive behavioral intervention for MS patients, researchers limited participants to those who met criteria regarding their gender, stage of disease, and degree of disability (Sinclair and Scroggie 2005). An established program with five sessions provided consistent intervention for study participants. Instruments were consistent and repeated measures were taken twice before the sessions began, immediately after completing the program, and six months following intervention. Everything about quantitative studies suggests that research follow a consistent plan to minimize the potential influence of outside events on study outcomes.

Contrast the methods reviewed in the quantitative study above with qualitative research methods. Qualitative research tends toward more fluid processes. Researchers select participants on the basis that they possess information about the phenomenon under study. To understand fully the broad aspects of the phenomenon, the study occurs in natural settings. Data, collected through semi-structured interviews, allows some variance between participants. The Barker-Collo et al. (2006) study of individuals living with MS selected participants to represent a broad spectrum of males and females with variable age ranges and times since diagnosis. Interview questions were open-ended and probe questions used to elicit further information. The processes of data collection and analysis flowed together and enabled study change. As new information became available through initial interviews and analysis, researchers were able to probe for more information in the new aspect identified and to redirect interview questions for future participants.

Scope

Scope refers to the amount of area that a study covers. Most quantitative studies have a relatively narrow scope because there is a need to exert control in the research setting. Investigators often use quantitative methods when something is already known about the phenomenon under study. Examine the summary of the quantitative study. Researchers here have narrowed the scope of the study to examine the effects of one particular type of intervention for women with MS. Even the title ("Effects of a Cognitive-Behavioral Program for Women with Multiple Sclerosis") gives readers a clue as to the scope of the study.

Compare this limited scope to that of a qualitative study about experiences of diagnosis and living with MS. Once again, the title ("Into the Unknown: The Experiences of Individuals Living with Multiple Sclerosis") offers some immediate insight into the possibility that the study has an expansive scope. In this example, you are comparing the quantitative results of a specific intervention to a wide range of experiences examined in the qualitative study.

Preconceptions

As researchers approach a quantitative study, they often are guided by a theoretical or conceptual framework. These preconceptions can influence their thinking about the outcomes of the study. For example, the researchers conducting the quantitative study used Lazarus and Folkman's Stress and Coping Model (1984), which influences the development of the cognitive behavioral intervention. Because of the Stress and Coping Model, researchers believe that they can influence the perceptions of women who have MS. These preconceptions extend to the development of the two study hypotheses.

In a quantitative study, hypotheses enable researchers to state what they anticipate the outcome of the study will be. In this instance, researchers predicted that patient perceptions of competence, coping, psychological well-being, quality of life, and fatigue levels would improve because of the intervention. Sinclair and Scroggie (2005) also proposed that these changes would be sustained or improved over the 6-month period following the intervention. Therefore, in quantitative studies, researchers clearly have preconceptions about the study outcomes even before the study begins.

Qualitative studies approach research quite differently. Very few preconceptions about the study outcome exist—and even if researchers have a preconceived idea, they try to ensure that those ideas do not influence their perspective about what participants are telling them. Notice in the qualitative study, the researchers state a broad purpose, but specific hypotheses are notably absent. Research is explorative in nature and investigators must be open to unexpected findings.

> ### Consider This . . .
> How do preconceptions differ from the actual hypothesis a researcher develops in a quantitative study?
> Researchers in qualitative studies may have preconceptions. How might researchers manage preconceptions to avoid influencing study outcomes?

Settings/Conditions

Research occurs in many different settings—in laboratories, in hospitals, and in communities. While each of these settings has advantages, control of the research setting and the conditions under which data are gathered are issues of concern. In order to prevent outside factors from influencing the outcome of the study, investigators conduct quantitative research in settings over which they can exert control.

Consistency in methods of sample selection, intervention, and measurement all work together to ensure that participants are treated similarly during data collection. It is easier to achieve high control in laboratory experiments. In social settings, quantitative researchers must take extra care to ensure consistency in settings and study methods. When studying the effects of a cognitive-behavioral intervention, Sinclair and Scroggie (2005) tried to control the research setting by specifying the type of individuals that would be included in their sample of 37 (diagnosis of relapsing-remitting MS, female gender, and a disability status score of under 6). To ensure consistency, participants received the same series of five weekly support groups and used a manual to facilitate practice of concepts taught in the support groups. Data collection used the same measures.

In contrast to the high-control settings found in quantitative research, qualitative research uses natural settings with few controls. Barker-Collo, Cartwright, and Read (2006) met participants (the word used in qualitative studies for research subjects) in their homes for a semi-structured interview. There was no intervention—investigators asked the 16 participants to share their experiences about diagnosis of their MS and the impact it had on their lives. However, it should be noted that qualitative research is not totally uncontrolled. Investigators tried to select a sample that reflected different backgrounds and times of diagnosis. They tried to select both male and female participants and had an evenly divided sample with participants diagnosed with relapsing-remitting MS and primary progressive MS.

Methods/Instruments

One of the most apparent differences in quantitative and qualitative research lies in the methods of data collection. Almost all studies—whether quantitative or qualitative—gather demographic (descriptive) information that is numerical in nature. However, beyond that point, methods become highly divergent. Quantitative studies gather information using instruments that lend themselves to numerical ratings. The Sinclair and Scroggie (2005) study measured each of the variables using quantitative instruments including but not limited to:

- Personal coping resources—The Perceived Health Competence Scale (8 items)
- Coping behavior—28-item Brief COPE
- Psychological well-being—5-item Satisfaction with Life Scale and a 20-item Positive and Negative Affect Schedule

Compare these quantitative instruments to those used in Barker-Collo, Cartwright, and Read's (2006) qualitative study, which used a semi-structured interview. Interviews invite participants to respond to broad, open-ended questions about their experiences, such as "describe the events that led up to receiving a diagnosis of MS" (p. 436). As the story unfolds, researchers may encourage the participant to elaborate on the details of the story. While most interviews ask a series of questions, researchers probe new areas if participants introduce them. The final product is narrative, usually captured on audiotape.

Some qualitative studies also use observation techniques. Sometimes researchers observe from an unobtrusive position or they serve in the role of a participant-observer who actively takes part in the setting while simultaneously collecting data. Once again, the investigators collect and record narrative information.

Analysis

The process of analysis also reveals differences between qualitative and quantitative research. First, examine the products of data collection. Quantitative researchers gather numerical information using scales and other quantitative measuring instruments, enter it into a database for analysis (often a computer software program), then interpret the findings. In Sinclair and Scroggins (2005) study of a cognitive behavioral intervention, many of the scales were given to subjects 4 times and were subsequently entered into a database for analysis. The specific analysis was determined for the hypothesis tested. At the end of the study, researchers compared the pretreatment scores on the instruments to the posttreatment scores to discover that participants experienced improvements following intervention in all of the areas except physical outcomes. Researchers also statistically compared the scores immediately following treatment to those 6 months later and found that participants sustained the improvements.

Compare a statistical analysis completed at the end of a quantitative study to the analysis the qualitative researchers give to the narrative materials they gathered. Instead of numbers, researchers must transcribe or type the taped interviews—usually verbatim—before they can begin the process of review. Analysis begins even as they transcribe. Analysis is usually time-consuming. Some investigators use a computer to organize and store information. In studies using observation where investigators recorded field notes, these notes are included in the analysis. Researchers sift through these narrative materials, looking both for common themes and for experiences that are markedly different from the rest of the group.

Note the methods used in the qualitative example: Analysis began early, after transcription of the first interview, and continued throughout the investigation. Investigators independently reviewed the transcripts to increase their familiarity. As they found similar information, they pulled out recurring themes and provided a descriptive label to the information. In this instance, investigators found thematic divisions to participants' processes of learning about and living with MS (prediagnosis, diagnosis, and reactions).

Note that both quantitative and qualitative analysis requires investigators to interpret the information they uncover. These interpretations are then discussed in light of the findings of other research and provide direction for new research proposals.

Thinking about Study Findings

So how would nurses caring for people with MS use the findings from these two different studies? The researchers who conducted the quantitative study learned several things useful to nurses:

- Lazarus and Folkman's (1984) theoretical framework, indicating that perceptions influence adaptation to stress, was correct. Individuals participating in the study felt more competent in caring for themselves and experienced greater psychological well-being that lasted even 6 months beyond the program.

- An intervention similar to the one used in the study is potentially useful for other women diagnosed with MS.

Nurses can use these quantitative study findings as a basis for developing an intervention for patients with MS. How does the broader ranging qualitative study about MS patients assist nurses in caring for their patients? Here, the findings relate to participant's early experiences as they received their MS diagnosis and offer nurses insight into patient perceptions regarding diagnosis:

- The study identified three phases associated with the process of MS diagnosis: the prediagnosis phase, actual diagnosis, and postdiagnosis. While participants recognized prediagnosis in hindsight, this phase, lasting over 5 years, was marked by confusion, anxiety, and uncertainty. Obtaining a diagnosis was an arduous process. Actual diagnosis brought a sense of relief but also uncertainty. The post diagnosis phase entailed not only dealing with chronic illness and uncertainty but also facing the discrimination and isolation generated by others' responses to illness.

- Timing of information delivery was critical because participants expressed that they were unable to process all of the information given and their information needs shifted over the course of disease.

Nurses can use these qualitative research findings in the following ways. First, nurses should be attentive to the uncertainty that occurs during all phases of an MS diagnosis. Nurses should consider information needs for patients and families and target information provision according to phase and the readiness of their patient to mentally process it. Inundating new MS patients with information at their diagnosis appointment does not serve patients well. Consider scheduling follow-up appointments targeted toward specific information needs. Be prepared to help patients and families work through post-diagnosis issues such as disease management, telling other people, and dealing with discrimination and isolation from others.

Michael Quinn Patton (2002) shares a parable about the process of discovery that helps to reflect the need for both quantitative and qualitative research. In his parable, a scholar who has read about fruit trees wants to experience what fruit is like. At the marketplace, he received explicit instructions about where to find the fruit trees and embarked on a journey of discovery. Following the instructions precisely, the scholar arrived at the orchard during springtime and found flowering apple trees. He pulled off the blossom and ate it only to find that it was bitter. So, he sampled another blossom with the same outcome. Although the blossoms were beautiful, he reported to his countrymen that fruit was overrated. The scholar never recognized the difference between the blossoms and the actual fruit that would grow in the summer. This parable demonstrates some differences in research methods. In this particular situation, the highly structured methods led to an erroneous outcome. Researchers must recognize the importance of choosing the method of discovery that best lends itself to the problem of study.

Consider This . . .

Which do you think uses a more scientific approach, quantitative or qualitative research? Why do you believe this to be true?

Of course, each method has value! In scientific discovery, the structured methods of quantitative research allow us to draw conclusions that are critical to discovering information that is generalizable to other groups. The trade-off is that the scope of studies may be very narrow, allowing researchers to miss the fact that flowers on an apple tree are not the fruit. Qualitative methods enable a broader focus of inquiry that helps investigators discover the seasons of the year and to pinpoint when fruit actually is edible. However, qualitative research does not have the ability for broad generalization to other groups and situations. For example, not all flowering trees bear edible fruit. Qualitative and quantitative research can complement one another. In many instances, qualitative discovery may offer direction to areas for quantitative study and theory testing. In other instances, quantitative findings may point to an area where more information is needed that would be best studied using in-depth qualitative methods. In order to continue discovery that is relevant to practice, nursing needs both quantitative and qualitative methods. This text explores both methods in greater depth so that you will readily recognize the nature of each research type and be able to evaluate its quality and usability in practice.

Ethical Considerations in Research

Human beings who participate in research studies provide substantial benefit for society. With this fact as a given, what responsibilities must researchers attend to in order to protect the rights of research participants? Regardless of the type of research conducted, investigators must consider the ethical aspects of conducting research to protect participants from potential harms.

History of Research Ethics

Prior to the middle of the 20th century, science did not specifically consider ethics of research to any great depth. However, when atrocities in biomedical research at German concentration camps were exposed following World War II, it led to the development of the Nuremberg Code (1949), a set of standards regarding the conduct of research. Unfortunately, atrocities such as these were not limited to wartime Germany. Numerous studies exploiting the rights of human subjects occurred in the United States. One of the most well-known examples, the Tuskegee Studies, still generates debate in research ethics circles (Brandt and Churchill 2000). Beginning in 1932, investigators observed 400 African-American men, mostly poor farmers, diagnosed with syphilis. Participants were never informed of their diagnosis other than being told that they had "bad blood," and were unaware of their enrollment in a research project (Reverby 2000, p. 1). This study, which lasted forty years, tracked participants to observe disease progression without ever offering treatment, even when penicillin became available in the 1940s. Although the study ended over 40 years ago, it powerfully symbolizes research gone awry and emphasizes the need for protections for human subjects.

In light of abuses occurring in research, in 1974 Congress passed the National Research Act, appointing a special commission known as the National Commission for the Protection of Human Subjects of Biomedical and Behavioral Research. This group of legal scholars, ethicists, researchers, and physicians composed a landmark report referred to as the Belmont Report (National Commission for the Protection of Human Subjects of Biomedical and Behavioral Research 1979). The **Belmont Report** helped to define the boundaries between therapy and research, and delineated three key ethical principles for consideration in the conduct of research using human subjects. Therapy is conceived as interventions done solely for the benefit of the person, whereas research treatments are done to assess outcomes in order to add to the scientific knowledge base.

An additional set of regulations called Title 45 Code of Federal Regulations Part 46 Protection of Human Subjects (45 CFR Part 46) provides a framework that must be used when engaging in research with human subjects (NIH 2005). These regulations encompass the principles offered by the Belmont Report and provide for a mechanism reviewing studies using human subjects. Update of these regulations continues to ensure protection for all human subjects.

Ethical Principles

The Belmont Report (National Commission for the Protection of Human Subjects of Biomedical and Behavioral Research 1979) delineated three ethical principles governing the conduct of research including respect for persons, beneficence, and justice. The principle **respect for persons** recognizes that individuals are autonomous human beings and have the capacity to make their own decisions. Another name sometimes used for this principle is respect for autonomy. Taking part in research requires that participants be informed about the nature of research and freely agree to be a part.

An important factor of respecting persons is special consideration for those who are vulnerable and lacking the capacity to fully and knowingly consent to research participation. Increased vulnerability for special groups of people occurs when they are ill, lack education, are poor, or lack the capacity to make decisions freely on their own behalf. In this situation, special safeguards must protect the interests of potential research participants.

Beneficence represents the second ethical consideration identified by the Belmont Report (1979). **Beneficence** has two areas to consider: first, to do no harm and second, to promote the welfare of individuals by maximizing the potential for benefit and minimizing the possibility for harm. This means that investigators must design studies minimizing the risk of harm to participating individuals. **Risk** is the likelihood that an injury or loss will occur in the future (Beauchamp and Childress 2009). It is not always possible to have risk-free research studies. Therefore, consideration of the benefits if the research is conducted enters into the picture. **Benefits** are those things that have a good effect, such as promoting well-being or avoiding costs (Beauchamp and Childress 2009). In research, investigators examine the risks of participating in a study in light of the benefits potentially gained. The Belmont Report (1979) warns that inhumane treatment cannot ever be justified and that risks should be minimized.

> **Consider This . . .**
>
> How much risk would be acceptable in a research study?

Justice is the third principle explored in the Belmont Report. **Justice** reflects the division of the benefits derived from research that are balanced against the burdens that such research might engender. How should these research benefits be distributed and who should bear the burden of research participation? Unfortunately, history demonstrates that the poor or least advantaged unfairly assume much of the burden of research while reaping few of the benefits. Consequently, researchers must consider issues of justice when selecting research subjects to ensure the fair distribution of benefits and burdens. For example, who should be enrolled in research studies? Must studies include men and women? Should children be enrolled? Are racial and ethnic minorities included? Which participants are the most appropriate for the protocol (U.S. Department of Health and Human Services 2004)?

Protection of Human Subjects

As the concerns and ethical principles in the Belmont Report and subsequent federal regulations developed to govern research make clear, research participants need protections to prevent abuse. Consequently, several processes have been put in place to review studies, ensure that risks and benefits of research participation are considered, facilitate informed consent, and protect the confidentiality of research participants.

INSTITUTIONAL REVIEW BOARDS. **Institutional Review Boards** (IRB) are groups that institutions such as universities or hospitals establish for the purpose of evaluating research proposals to ensure that federal guidelines for human subject protection are met (Protection of Human Subjects 2005). Operating under federal regulations, these bodies have authority to review studies and require modifications prior to permitting the study to move forward. IRBs strive to minimize the risks associated with a study and put adequate safeguards in place. When risks exist, IRBs consider the potential benefits derived from conducting the research. IRBs also try to ensure the selection of research participants is equitable: that special groups are not excluded nor any group singled out to assume undue risk.

INFORMED CONSENT. Based on the ethical principle of respect for persons, investigators must consider decisions autonomous people make regarding their willingness to participate in a study. **Informed consent** is a statement that describes the proposed research, including the purpose of the study, what participants will do, the length of time participation will take, and the potential risks of taking part (Protection of Human Subjects 2005). In other words, before a person enrolls in a research study, they must give their permission based on details of the study. Consent information is organized and written in such a way that all potential participants can understand it. Agreement to participate must be voluntary and not have penalties attached when people decline participation. A specific function of IRBs is to review informed consents to ensure that they meet guidelines for adequately informing participants. The accompanying *Research in the News* box underscores the need for informed consent in research.

Individuals lacking the capacity to make their own decisions require special protection. For example, parents or a guardian must consent to research participation for children or for adults lacking capacity to give their own informed consent. Parent or guardian consent does not necessarily relieve investigators from asking the potential subject about their willingness to participation. In many instances the parent or guardian must give the official research consent, but the actual participant must assent or agree to be a part of the research as well. **Assent** is the agreement of a child or person lacking capacity to participate in research. When the parent or guardian consents *and* the child or adult lacking capacity assents, study participation may begin.

CONFIDENTIALITY. When research information is collected from individuals, an important issue is confidentiality. **Confidentiality** suggests that when one person divulges information to another person or group, the information will be kept private unless explicit permission is given for information release (Beauchamp and Childress 2009). In research, confidentiality of information is a significant concern. Research participants may be reluctant to share personal information unless they have assurances that the information will not be identifiable. Research strategies employed to protect confidentiality include using code numbers to identify collected data rather than participant names, storing raw research data in password-protected computers, and reporting pooled data that does not identify

Research in the News

Lawsuits Settled over Arizona Tribe Blood Samples

BY AMANDA LEE MYERS
Associated Press, April 21, 2010

PHOENIX — An Arizona Indian tribe has ended a seven-year legal fight over blood samples members gave to university scientists for diabetes research that were later used to study schizophrenia, inbreeding and ancient population migration in what tribal members called a case of genetic piracy.

The Havasupai Indians, who live deep in a gorge off the Grand Canyon, settled their lawsuits with Arizona State University in an agreement announced Wednesday and approved by the Legislature's Joint Legislative Budget Committee on Tuesday.

The Havasupai claimed ASU conducted the additional research without permission, invading tribal members' privacy, betraying the tribe's trust and misrepresenting what researchers had done with blood samples and subsequent research results.

The settlement includes a lump $700,000 payment to the 41 plaintiffs, and the university has agreed to help the tribe seek third-party funding to build a new health clinic and high school in the isolated village. ASU also has agreed to give the tribe the more than 200 blood samples, which members say will be buried in a sacred ceremony, some with the remains of the people who gave the blood.

"Their spirits will no longer be locked in a cooler," said Carletta Tilousi, the lead

plaintiff in the case and a tribal council woman. "We are going to take them back down to Supai Canyon so they can rest in peace."

Tilousi, most of her family members and other tribal members gave their blood to scientists in the 1990s thinking it would be used to help cure diabetes.

The research was requested by Tilousi's aunt, who was on dialysis and had to have a leg amputated because of diabetes before her death last year.

The research concluded that diabetes among the tribe was not related to genetics.

Tribal officials complained in 2003 after learning of the additional research and filed lawsuits after they weren't satisfied when they met with university representatives. The tribe had asked for $50 million in its pre-litigation claim. Individuals who filed the other separate lawsuit sought $10 million.

Ernest Calderon, president of the Arizona Board of Regents, said in a statement that the board "has long wanted to remedy the wrong that was done."

"This solution is not simply the end of a dispute but is also the beginning of a partnership between the universities, principally ASU and the tribe."

Tilousi said she hoped the settlement would make a statement on behalf of all indigenous people that their cultures should be respected, not analyzed by scientists.

continued. . .

> *Havasupai Chairwoman Bernadine Jones said the settlement "is far more than dismissing a lawsuit."*   *"The settlement is the restoration of hope for my people, and the beginning of nation building for my tribe," she said.*

Read the headline news report concerning ethical issues related to conducting research.

What ethical issue is at the center of the dispute between the Havasupai Indians and the scientists studying blood samples from the tribe?

A key sentence about the claim is:

The Havasupai claimed ASU conducted the additional research without permission, invading tribal members' privacy, betraying the tribe's trust and misrepresenting what researchers had done with blood samples and subsequent research results.

This sentence tells us that researchers did not get consent for further study on blood samples.

Consider whether or not the Havasupai tribal members are justified in feeling mistrustful of researchers because of the additional uses of their blood samples.

Should scientists have the right to conduct research on blood samples or body tissues in ways that were not included in the original consent? Why or why not?

The full story can be found at: Meyers, A.L. 2010. Lawsuits settled over Arizona tribe blood samples. *Houston Chronicle*. Retrieved from http://www.chron.com /disp/story.mpl/nation/6969619.html

---

Resource and Subject Matter

specific individuals. A research term that is closely related to confidentiality is anonymity. **Anonymity** refers to information that has no identifying features that would potentially link a participant to the research study. Anonymity is different from confidentiality. With anonymous data, even the researcher could not identify the participant. With confidential data, researchers can identify the participant, but take action to avoid revealing participant identity to anyone else. IRBs review research applications to ensure that safeguards are in place to protect identifiable data and that consent forms clearly explain the extent to which research information is confidential (U.S. Department of Health and Human Services 2004).

Scientific Misconduct

Research findings are credible because we depend on the integrity of investigators to plan and conduct sound studies. We anticipate that those involved with research are honest and straightforward as they collect, analyze, and interpret data as well as when findings are reported. Unfortunately, in some instances, a few researchers manipulate the outcomes of a study or misrepresent the study findings. **Scientific misconduct** "means fabrication, falsification, plagiarism, or other practices that seriously deviate from those that are commonly accepted within the scientific community for proposing, conducting, or reporting research. It does not include honest error or honest differences in interpretations or judgments of data" (Handling Misconduct 1989, § 50.102). Fabrication implies researchers made up data while falsification implies changing data outcomes. Plagiarism reflects stealing work by copying someone else's words or ideas without giving credit to the source. All of these activities are wrong and subsequently affect the credibility of research outcomes. To ensure that studies are properly conducted, oversight for research is provided by institutions and by the Office of Research Integrity, a federal agency that is part of the U.S. Department of Health and Human Services. The oversight process helps people feel that scientific findings represent credible research processes.

SUMMARY

In this chapter we discussed the differences between quantitative and qualitative research and ethical issues all research must consider.

- Two major philosophical orientations influence our conceptions about what truth is and how to best discover the way **phenomena** work. **Positivism** states that a reality exists which is best discovered through a systematic series of highly controlled quantitative studies, while **constructivism** proposes that multiple realities exist and that these realities are mediated by experiences. *(Objective 1)*

- Quantitative and qualitative research reflect different approaches for planning and structuring studies. **Quantitative research** tends to have a tightly defined scope, gathering information using measurement techniques that permit numeric calculation under situations of high control. **Qualitative research** tends to have a broader scope and information is collected in more naturalistic settings. It focuses on collecting and analyzing narrative data. *(Objective 2)*

- Prior to World War II there was very little regulation of research using human subjects. Subsequent to many abuses, regulations to protect individuals participating in research were enacted, including the Nuremburg Code and federal regulations as recommended by the **Belmont Report**. *(Objective 3)*

- Three major ethical principles guide the conduct of research: **respect for persons**, which recognizes the rights of individuals to make decisions, **beneficence**, which weighs potential risks and benefits of research in order to protect research subjects from harm, and **justice**, which is concerned with balancing the distribution of the benefits and burdens of research. *(Objective 4)*

- Hospitals, schools, and other institutions appoint **Institutional Review Boards** (IRBs) to evaluate research protocols and ensure sound science and safety of proposed research studies. **Informed consent** is the process whereby potential research subjects are given information regarding the purpose of research studies, the nature of interventions that subject will receive, and the risks that are present in the study. **Scientific misconduct** occurs when researchers fabricate or falsify data or plagiarize the ideas or words of others. Federal regulations codify safeguards to ensure that studies are conducted correctly. *(Objective 5)*

STUDENT ACTIVITIES

1. Find a research article that is related to clinical practice.
    - What problem does the article address?
    - Is the study approach quantitative or qualitative?
    - What procedures did the researchers use to gather information?
    - How might nurses use the findings in this study?

2. **Hot Topic Discussion:** You are a student in a nursing education program.
   - How would you respond if you felt coerced into participating in an educational study?
   - Discuss ethical principles or protections that should be considered in recruiting study participants.

3. You are a research nurse getting consent for a study. Develop a list of questions about a study that would need to be answered before consent could be given.

4. Examine the newspaper or a news web site for stories about health care research. How useful is the information in these stories for the public? How useful is the information for health care professionals?

Pearson Nursing Student Resources
Find additional review materials at
www.nursing.pearsonhighered.com
Prepare for success with additional NCLEX®-style practice questions, interactive assignments and activities, web links, animations and videos, and more!

REFERENCES

Barker-Collo, S., C. Cartwright, and J. Read. 2006. Into the unknown: The experiences of individuals living with multiple sclerosis. *Journal of Neuroscience Nursing, 38*(6): 435–441, 446.

Beauchamp, T. and J. Childress. 2009. *Principles of biomedical ethics.* (6th ed.) New York, NY: Oxford University Press.

Brandt, A. and L. Churchill. 2000. Preface. In S. Reverby (Ed.), *Tuskegee truths: Rethinking the Tuskegee syphilis study,* (pp. xv–xvi). Chapel Hill, NC: University of North Carolina Press.

Guba, E.G. and Y.S. Lincoln. 1994. Competing paradigms in qualitative research. In E.K. Dentin & Y.S. Lincoln (Eds.), *Handbook of qualitative research,* (pp. 105–117). Thousand Oaks, CA: Sage. (p. 109, 112).

Handling Misconduct, Title 42 CFR, Part 50. 1989. Retrieved from http://ori.dhhs.gov/misconduct/reg_subpart_a.shtml

Lazarus, R. and S. Folkman. 1984. *Stress, appraisal, and coping.* New York, NY: Springer.

Meyers, A.L. 2010. Lawsuits settled over Arizona tribe blood samples. *Houston Chronicle.* Retrieved from http://www.chron.com/disp/story.mpl/nation/6969619.html

National Commission for the Protection of Human Subjects of Biomedical and Behavioral Research.
1979. *The Belmont report: Ethical principles and guidelines for the protection of human subjects of research.* Retrieved from http://ohsr.od.nih.gov/guidelines/belmont.html

Nuremberg Code. 1949. *Trials of War Criminals before the Nuremberg Military Tribunals under Control Council Law No. 10,* Vol. 2, pp. 181–182. Washington, DC: U.S. government Printing Office. Retrieved from http://ohsr.od.nih.gov/guidelines/nuremberg.html

Patton, M.Q. 2002. *Qualitative research and evaluation methods* (3rd ed.). Thousand Oaks, CA: Sage.

Protection of Human Subjects, Title 45 CFR, Part 46. 2005. Retrieved from http://ohsr.od.nih.gov/guidelines/45cfr46.html

Reverby, S. 2000. *Tuskegee truths: Rethinking the Tuskegee syphilis study.* Chapel Hill, NC: University of North Carolina Press.

Sinclair, V. and J. Scroggie. 2005. Effects of a cognitive-behavioral program for women with multiple sclerosis. *Journal of Neuroscience Nursing, 37*(5): 249–257, 276.

U.S. Department of Health and Human Services, National Institutes of Health. 2004. *Guidelines for the conduct of research involving human subjects* (NIH Publication No. 00-4783). Retrieved from http://ohsr.od.nih.gov/guidelines/GrayBooklet82404.pdf.

The Quantitative Research Process

CHAPTER OUTLINE

CHAPTER OBJECTIVES

1. Discuss the integration of the phases and steps of the quantitative research process.
2. Examine the steps in conceptualizing the research problem.
3. Examine the steps involved in designing a quantitative research study.
4. Examine the steps involved in implementing a quantitative study design.
5. Examine the steps involved in analyzing and interpreting data from a quantitative study.
6. Explore the use of quantitative study findings in nursing practice.

KEY TERMS

Conceptual definition (**p. 83**)
Conceptual framework (**p. 81**)
Control (**p. 83**)
Data (**p. 91**)
Dependent variable (**p. 83**)
Descriptive statistics (**p. 98**)
Dissemination (**p. 103**)
Extraneous variable (**p. 83**)
Findings (**p. 102**)
Generalizability (**p. 89**)
Hypothesis (**p. 84**)

Implication (**p. 103**)
Independent variable (**p. 83**)
Instruments (**p. 91**)
Literature review (**p. 80**)
Non-probability sample (**p. 89**)
Operational definition (**p. 84**)
Population (**p. 88**)
Probability sample (**p. 89**)
Problem statement (**p. 78**)
Purpose (**p. 78**)
Quantitative research (**p. 77**)

Reliability (**p. 92**)
Research design (**p. 86**)
Research problem (**p. 77**)
Research question (**p. 84**)
Sample (**p. 88**)
Sampling (**p. 88**)
Setting (**p. 88**)
Theoretical framework (**p. 80**)
Theory (**p. 81**)
Validity (**p. 93**)
Variables (**p. 83**)

ABSTRACT

Quantitative research is a systematic, objective process of posing questions about variables and the relationships among variables and then measuring and testing those relationships using precise statistical methods. The quantitative research process uses a precise series of phases and steps to conduct an inquiry about an identified research problem.

In Phase 1, Conceptualize the Problem, *a conceptual foundation is formed. The problem is identified, the literature is reviewed, a theoretical frame of reference is developed, and research questions or hypotheses are formulated. In Phase 2,* Design the Study, *a plan for the conduct of the study is devised. A research design is chosen; a setting, sample, and sampling technique are adopted; and instruments are selected and examined for reliability and validity. Phase 3,* Implement the Design, *entails consideration of participant rights, participant recruitment and retention, and data collection. Phase 4,* Analyze the Data, *involves describing the sample, answering the research questions/hypotheses, and interpreting the results. Phase 5,* Use the Results, *is the final phase and involves the dissemination of the results by the researcher and the use of the results by the practicing nurse.*

This chapter examines the phases and steps involved in the quantitative research process in detail. We will define quantitative research and investigate key concepts that are critical to your understanding of the phases and steps of the quantitative research process. This chapter will further expand your research vocabulary and will prove useful as we examine actual research studies and their application to your nursing practice in the chapters to come.

Overview of Quantitative Research

Recall from Chapter 4 that quantitative research involves the systematic collection and analysis of numerical information. The quantitative researcher uses precise instruments that allow the collection and conversion of data into numerical form. These numbers can then be subjected to statistical analysis. Adding to that description, we can conceptualize **quantitative research** as a systematic, objective process used to pose questions about variables and the relationships among variables and then to measure and test those relationships using precise statistical methods. The process starts at a beginning point (asking a question) and moves in a fairly linear sequence to an end point (obtaining an answer). The process used is remarkably similar for all quantitative studies. Some steps may overlap or be unnecessary but generally the phases and steps form a pattern that is readily identified with the quantitative tradition.

Quantitative Research Process

We examined the five phases of the research process in Chapter 3. Now we are going to examine that process for quantitative research. You will note a series of steps inherent to each of the five phases have now been added to the model. Figure 5-1 illustrates the phases and steps of the research process.

Phase 1: Conceptualize the Problem

There are four major steps in the conceptualization phase. The researcher searches and analyzes the existing literature, articulates a problem, refines and places it in a theoretical context, and identifies and defines the study variables. Problem formulation, review of the literature, and theoretical contextualization often occur concurrently and ultimately lead to the identification and definition of variables to be studied.

Formulate the Problem

The first task that a researcher confronts is to identify and describe the problem to be studied. A **research problem** originates from a situation in which people recognize that unsolved difficulties exist. It is a "felt need"—a gap in the knowledge base. That need might arise from a particular concern in one's own nursing practice or it might come from deficiencies in the published literature such as contradictory reports or untested opinions or conclusions. The literature represents the current state of nursing science. It influences the ways that nurses practice by providing evidence to guide that practice. Thus, gaps in the literature can affect practice. Researchers search for those gaps and attempt to fill them to advance the state of the science.

Consider This . . .

What needs, if any, have you noticed in your clinical experiences that you think would benefit from research?

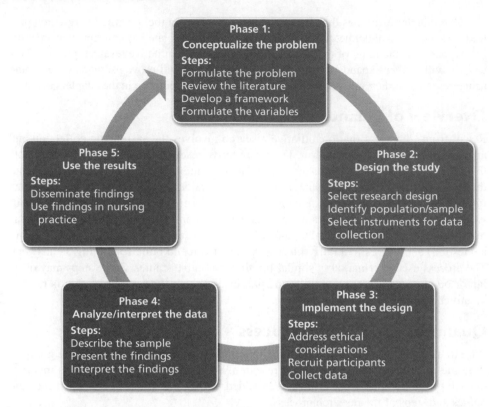

■ FIGURE 5-1 **The Quantitative Research Process**
(Adapted from Langford 2001)
Note the expansion of the figure from Chapter 3. Now each phase has specific steps delineated for that phase.

The problem is articulated as a **problem statement**, a one or two paragraph discussion that describes the problem, provides background and significance for the problem, and states a rationale that supports the need for a study of the problem. It tells us what, who, and why. Researchers also describe the study's **purpose**, which reveals the intent or goal of the study. This might be expressed as a purpose, an aim, or an objective. This statement may also describe the type or classification of the study and usually provides more specificity to the concepts of interest.

Box 5-1 contains examples of problem statements and purpose statements. Note in Example 1 that the problem is described as music effects on stress. It also identifies patients on ventilators as the targeted group of interest. The need for the study is stated as a gap in the currently available literature. The use of the term *pilot study* in the purpose tells us that this is a preliminary look at the problem. It also states that biomarkers will be used to examine the stress response. In Example 2, the problem is described as illness and physical limitations that could be prevented by physical activity. The group of interest is rural adults in small towns. The study is needed because few studies have looked at this problem for people in rural areas. The purpose is to test the effects of telephone only motivational interviewing (MI) intervention to see whether it increases physical activity.

> **BOX 5-1** Sample Problem Statement and Purpose
>
> **Example 1: Influence of music on the stress response in patients receiving mechanical ventilatory support: a pilot study**
>
> **Problem Statement**
>
> "Music is one nonpharmacological intervention that is considered an ideal therapy for reducing stress in patients receiving mechanical ventilatory support.1 Music affects indirect markers of activity of the sympathetic nervous system (SNS) in these patients, as evidenced by reductions in heart rate, respiratory rate, and blood pressure. The central nervous system, however, has 2 main components involved in the stress response: the hypothalamic-pituitary adrenal (HPA) axis and the SNS. Previous research on the effects of music in patients receiving mechanical ventilation has focused solely on indirect markers of SNS activity. Little evidence has been collected about music's influence on biomarkers that reflect activity of both components involved in the stress response" (Chlan et al. 2007, p. 141).
>
> **Purpose**
>
> "The purpose of this pilot study was to explore the influence of music on serum levels of biomarkers of the stress response in patients receiving ventilatory support" (Chlan et al. 2007, p. 141).
>
> **Example 2: A telephone-only motivational intervention to increase physical activity in rural adults: A randomized controlled trial**
>
> **Problem Statement**
>
> "Physical inactivity has been called a silent epidemic in the United States accounting for an increasing incidence of many chronic illnesses, including cancer. Although the health hazards of inactivity are known, few Americans meet national recommendations for daily physical activity, and rural adults, in particular, are very inactive. Rural adults have higher rates of chronic illness and physical limitations that might be prevented by increased physical activity yet few studies have been focused on helping people increase their regular physical activity in rural environments" (Bennett et al. 2008, p. 24).
>
> **Purpose**
>
> "The purpose of this study was to evaluate whether a telephone-only MI intervention, delivered from one location by a physical activity counselor trained in MI, would increase the physical activity of rural adults in small towns in a broad geographic area" (Bennett et al. 2008, p. 25).

When formulating a research problem and purpose, researchers must keep several considerations in mind. They must ensure that the selected problem be researchable, significant, and feasible. The most important consideration is whether the ideas chosen for study can be clearly defined and measured and whether the answer matters to nursing. If so, the problem is researchable and significant. Keep in mind that not all problems are researchable. For example, research cannot deal with moral or ethical problems, so the research process is not appropriate to consider issues such as whether abortion is murder or whether euthanasia should be legal. Instead, research focuses on those things that can be observed and/or measured. This entails consideration of researcher interest and expertise, availability of resources, and ethical concerns. The researcher or research team needs prior knowledge of and experience in the area that will be investigated as well as familiarity with the research process. Researcher interest and enthusiasm for the chosen problem is also important. Carrying out research for an identified problem can be a long and complex process that requires a considerable investment of time and energy. A passion for the study provides energy for the persistence to see the study through.

Consideration of resources includes an examination of a number of factors. These include aspects such as time, participants, facilities, personnel, supplies, equipment, and possible funding resources. When considering time, the researcher must look at whether the scope of the chosen problem has been narrowed enough to be studied in the time allotted. The researcher also needs to consider whether there are enough potential study participants and a means to access those potential participants and associated facilities. Projected expenses (personnel, equipment, and supplies) need to be identified as this will allow the researcher to determine what funds are necessary to carry out the research.

The researcher must also examine whether the problem proposed for study is feasible from an ethics standpoint. This means that researchers must be familiar with the ethical principles that must be considered when designing any research study to ensure that the rights of potential participants will not be violated. These ethical principles are discussed in Chapter 4.

Review the Literature

Quantitative researchers search existing literature to better understand what is already known about the research that they propose to conduct. As we explored in Chapter 2, the **literature review** involves a search for information that is relevant to the identified problem area and reveals how the problem fits into the larger picture of evidence and in what context. This results in a critical summary of the knowledge that exists and highlights any gaps in that knowledge about the problem of interest. This also serves to assist in clarifying and honing the research problem and allows the current research to build smoothly on an existing foundation. The review is also useful in developing and refining the theoretical frame of reference (the third step of Phase 1).

A good literature review possesses several key characteristics. It should be comprehensive, relevant, and balanced. In other words, it should cover all the current theoretical and research content on the concepts that have been identified in the problem statement and purpose. *Relevancy* refers to whether the sources have a direct bearing on the identified problem. Balance is achieved by ensuring that the scope of the review is broad enough to familiarize the reader with the problem area and narrow enough to focus on core information provided primarily by research studies as opposed to theoretical narratives. *Balance* also means that the review includes studies that may not support the researcher's preconceived notions.

You might want to review the procedures and databases used to conduct a literature review discussed in Chapter 2. Researchers engage in this systematic search process when reviewing the available literature. The review of literature in a published research study is typically presented in abbreviated form. The goals in such a review are twofold: to provide the reader with a snapshot of the existing knowledge on the topic under study and to provide support that the proposed research is necessary and fills an identified gap in the current literature.

Develop a Framework

A **theoretical framework** uses a theory or theories to form a frame of reference for the research study. This foundation both gives a rationale for the study and provides a conceptual basis for the study. This theoretical foundation in turn allows the researcher to link eventual study outcomes to the existing body of knowledge that was uncovered during the literature review. Placing study results in the larger context of relevant literature gives the findings greater utility and allows them to be more broadly applied to everyday settings.

A **theory** consists of a number of well-integrated and interrelated concepts used to explain some phenomenon. The concepts and many of the relationships have been previously tested and researched. Theories help nurse researchers pull complex concepts together. They demonstrate how these concepts interact and function as a larger whole. This allows us to more effectively order knowledge, thus increasing understanding of the bigger picture. Whether you realize it or not, you already use a number of theories that have been introduced in the course of your education. Nursing has long pulled theories from related disciplines such as sociology, psychology, and the biomedical sciences. Does Selye's theory of stress, Piaget's theory of development, or Pasteur's germ theory sound familiar? What about the theories explaining phenomena such as homeostasis, immunity, or pain? We apply such theories every day in the course of our clinical practice. Nurses have also developed a number of theories to explain nursing practice. Our practice of nursing has been built on the theorizing of such nursing greats as Hildegard Peplau, Martha Rogers, Imogene King, Sister Callista Roy, and Dorothea Orem.

A clearly identified framework is one indication of a well-conceived study. This is important because the relationship of theory, research, and practice is a circular one. Theories support and serve as a foundation for research problems. Research results confirm or refute theory explanations. This in turn allows the theory to be revised or fine-tuned, which then provides future avenues for research. Theories also guide practice and allow us to be more efficient and effective in that practice. Practice in turn points up weaknesses in theory and helps to further shape and mold theory. Research is the ultimate key in the development of nursing as a discipline. As the state of nursing science evolves, the use and refinement of theory and the application of theory to professional practice grows. Note that research, theory, and practice interact with each other in a reciprocal, cyclical manner (Figure 5-2).

When research in an area is new or preliminary, a conceptual rather than a theoretical approach may be used when forming a framework for the study. A **conceptual framework**

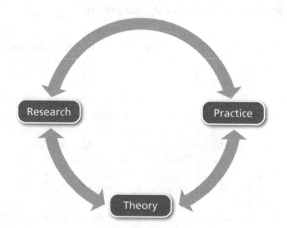

■ **FIGURE 5-2** Cycle of Research, Theory, and Practice
Research, theory, and practice constantly interact with one another reciprocally and cyclically.

is similar to a theoretical framework. However, in conceptual frameworks, the structure is less formally organized, concepts are more loosely related, and links between concepts have yet to be meaningfully tested. The theoretical or conceptual framework may be illustrated graphically through the use of a model. A picture or graphic is often a powerful way to illustrate concepts and their relationships at a glance. An example of a model can be seen in Figure 5-2. This particular model illustrates the way that research, theory, and practice are linked.

Not all research studies use an expressly described framework, but all studies use some type of implied framework or theoretical rationale. If a study does not clearly state the framework, however, it leaves the reader to wonder what the researchers had in mind when conducting the study. The lack of a clearly articulated framework also makes it harder to integrate research results back into the current body of knowledge.

Box 5-2 illustrates the frameworks used in the examples of problem statements and purposes from the two studies that we viewed in Box 5-1. The framework in the first example is alluded to very briefly: the study uses a physiologic stress response theory as the framework and zeroes in on the HPA and SNS components of this theory. The second example spells out the framework in one sentence and states clearly that the study is based on two theoretical influences, Prochaska's transtheoretical model of health behavior and Bandura's social cognitive theory. It then goes on to discuss how the MI intervention being tested in the study fits into the selected theoretical framework.

BOX 5-2 Examples of Theoretical Frameworks

Example 1: Influence of music on the stress response in patients receiving mechanical ventilatory support: a pilot study

Framework
"The central nervous system, however, has 2 main components involved in the stress response: the hypothalamic-pituitary adrenal (HPA) axis and the SNS" (Chlan et al. 2007, p. 141).

Example 2: A telephone-only motivational intervention to increase physical activity in rural adults: A randomized controlled trial

Framework
"One such intervention is motivational interviewing (MI), based on the transtheoretical model of health behavior change (Prochaska & Velicer, 1997) and social cognitive theory (Bandura, 1977, 1986)" (Bennett et al. 2008, p. 24).

"Motivational interviewing is a client-centered counseling procedure that includes four major strategies to help clients move toward behavior change: (a) expressing empathy, (b) supporting self-efficacy, (c) rolling with resistance, and (d) developing discrepancy between current behaviors and desired behaviors. The goal is to help clients express their own barriers to change, to explore how their current health behavior may conflict with their own goals and values, and to choose how to work on behavior change. . . . A key concept of MI is that individuals' self-efficacy or belief that they can accomplish a behavior change is a predictor of treatment outcome (Miller & Rollnick, 2002). Perceived self-efficacy, derived from the framework of social cognitive theory and incorporated into MI, refers to individuals' belief that they can organize and carry out actions, an essential component of undertaking a new activity and continuing to engage in that activity (Bandura, 1977, 1986)." (Bennett et al. 2008, p. 25).

Formulate the Variables

Variables are identified attributes or concepts that vary or change. These attributes are typically associated with persons, groups, or situations. Almost any concept or attribute that varies and can be observed and measured may be considered a variable. For example, gender, race, marital status, height, and weight are all attributes that vary from person to person. Variables are key building blocks in quantitative research. Research studies are specifically designed to measure, manipulate, or control variables.

Variables may take different forms. They may be classified by quality or quantity. Qualitative or categorical variables are variables that change in terms of the presence or absence of a specified attribute (e.g. male or not male, married or not married). Quantitative variables are variables that change in terms of amount or degree (e.g. height expressed in inches or weight measured in pounds). These variables can be described in precise numbers and fractions of numbers. This qualitative or quantitative classification becomes an important issue when selecting the appropriate statistics to find an answer to the research problem.

Another way to classify variables is to determine whether a particular variable is acting as an independent variable, a dependent variable, or an extraneous variable in a research study. The **independent variable** is the variable that is used to explain or predict the change or variation in the **dependent variable**. The dependent variable is also known as the outcome variable. For example, in a study that is researching whether "an omega 3 enriched diet" will improve heart health by decreasing "C-reactive protein levels," the "type of diet" is the independent variable and the "levels of C-reactive protein in the blood" is the dependent variable. The independent variable can be considered the cause, while the dependent variable is the effect.

Extraneous variables are other variables that can affect the dependent variable and interfere with the relationship of the independent and dependent variables. In the example above, extraneous variables such as "exercise" or "weight" or "gum inflammation" might also affect "C-reactive protein levels."

Consider This . . .

How can you tell if a variable is extraneous?

Researchers try to identify all of the variables that might have an impact on the dependent variable. They can then **control** those identified extraneous variables and keep them from interfering with the relationships between the independent variables and dependent variables that they are interested in studying. The literature review helps researchers to identify these extraneous factors. A number of methods can be used to exert control over these extraneous factors once they are identified. For example, the way that researchers select samples, assign samples to groups, or choose statistical techniques can all be used to help control extraneous variables.

Once variables are identified, they must be defined. Variables are defined in two ways. The first is a **conceptual definition**. This is the type of definition that you are familiar with and is the abstract or theoretical meaning of the variable. This definition is derived from a review of the theoretical literature and is used to place the meaning of the variable in the given context of the research study. The definition of the term *research* found on page 45, Chapter 3 serves as an excellent example of a conceptual definition.

The second definition is an **operational definition**. This definition spells out how the variable will be measured or manipulated in a research study. For example, the variable "pain" might be conceptually defined as "an unpleasant sensory and emotional experience associated with actual or potential tissue damage" (IASP 1994). The operational definition might state that "pain" will be measured using a visual analog pain rating scale.

In a specific research study, variables come from the concepts identified in the problem statement or purpose and can specified either in the form of research questions or hypotheses. **Research questions** identify the variables under study and ask how those variables might be described and/or what differences or relationships exist between those variables. Research questions should also identify who is being studied. Box 5-3 shows examples of research questions from actual studies. In the first example, the researchers want to identify differences between two groups. The independent variable is whether or not the participants attended camp. The dependent variable is QOL (quality of life). Adolescents with diabetes are the identified participants. The second example illustrates a slightly different approach as the researchers want to describe the actions of one variable. Both research questions seek to describe the time interval between event A and event B. Thus the variable of interest in this study is the time interval.

BOX 5-3 Sample Research Questions

Example 1: A study by Cheung et al. (2006) that examined quality of life in Diabetic adolescents who went to camp asked the following research question: "Is QOL in adolescents with diabetes who attend diabetes camp higher than the QOL in adolescents with diabetes who have never attended diabetes camp?" (p. 54)

Example 2: A study by Cohen et al. (2007) that examined diabetes management in an acute care setting posed the following research questions:

1. "What is the interval of time between morning capillary blood glucose monitoring and injection of short acting insulin? (p. 486)
2. What is the interval of time between morning capillary blood glucose monitoring and breakfast time?" (p. 486)

Consider This . . .

How would you reframe the research need you identified from your clinical practice and state it in the form of a research question?

A **hypothesis**, on the other hand, makes a prediction about the expected outcomes of the study. It is an educated guess about the relationship or differences among certain identified variables based on information found in the literature review and the links seen among concepts in the selected theoretical framework. When researchers don't have enough information to state a hypothesis, they instead pose a research question. When variables are clearly identified in the purpose statement, a study may forgo the hypotheses or research questions altogether.

All hypotheses contain at least one identifiable independent variable and at least one dependent variable. Such hypotheses are labeled as simple hypotheses. When a hypothesis contains more than one independent or more than one dependent variable, it is called a complex hypothesis. Hypotheses should also identify the participants in the study.

If you look at Box 5-4 you will see that Example 1 tests two hypotheses in one study. Both of these hypotheses are classified as simple hypotheses as they contain one independent variable and one dependent variable. In both hypotheses, the independent variable is the type of nursing intervention (use of case management versus use of assessment and information card). The dependent variable in the first hypothesis is safety behaviors and the dependent variable in the second hypothesis is use of community resources. The study participants are abused women.

Example 2 also shows two hypotheses. Let's examine the first hypothesis. The independent variable here is the presence or absence of IBS. The dependent variables are stress and psychological distress. As you can see, the researchers are making a prediction that women with IBS are more stressed and distressed than women who do not have IBS. So the presence or absence of IBS (independent variable) is projected to influence the degree of stress and distress (dependent variables). Because there are two dependent variables stated in this hypothesis, it would be classified as a complex hypothesis. In the second hypothesis, the dependent variables are severity of abdominal discomfort and bowel pattern symptoms. The independent variable is intensity level of stress. In this hypothesis, the intensity of stress (independent variable) is expected to influence the severity of discomfort and bowel patterns. The presence of two dependent variables also classifies this as a complex hypothesis. The study participants are women.

BOX 5-4 Examples of Simple and Complex Hypotheses

Example 1
A study by McFarlane et al. (2006) that focused on prevention of intimate partner violence tested the following hypotheses:

1. "Abused women who participate in the nurse case management intervention will report more adopted safety behaviors than abused women who receive abuse assessment and an information card only.

2. Abused women who participate in the nurse case management intervention will report greater use of community resources than abused women who receive abuse assessment and an information card only". (p. 2)

Example 2
A study by Hertig et al. (2008) that focused on stress and GI symptoms in women with IBS tested the following hypotheses:

1. "Women with IBS will report higher levels of stress and psychological distress compared with women without IBS.

2. Intensity of stress will be associated with severity of abdominal discomfort symptoms and bowel pattern symptoms." (p. 400)

Key:
Independent variables
Dependent variables

The hypothesis crystallizes the conceptualization of the research undertaken in Phase 1. This phase lays the conceptual and theoretical foundation for the research study. When done well, the research rests on a firm foundation. When this phase is not well thought out, the study is built on shifting sand which can make the findings of such a study questionable.

Phase 2: Design the Study

In Phase 2, researchers decide about the methods and procedures they will use to find the answers to the research problem identified in Phase 1. There are three major steps in this phase: selecting the research design, identifying the population and sample, and choosing the best instrument for collecting the data. While Phase 1 focused on abstract and conceptual thought, this phase focuses on the mechanics of the study.

Select the Research Design

The **research design** is the overall plan that guides the way the study is conducted. There are two major categories of quantitative research design: experimental and non-experimental. One important factor separates experimental from non-experimental designs. In an experimental study, the researcher is interested in whether the independent variable is causing the effect on the dependent variable. To test this cause and effect relationship, the researcher actively manipulates the independent variable in an attempt to create a change in the dependent variable. This manipulation is also known as a treatment or an intervention. In a non-experimental study, the researcher collects data on the identified variables but no intervention is administered by the researcher. Explore the *Research in the News* box. It speaks to research design.

Research in the News

Low-Salt Diet Ineffective, Study Finds. Disagreement Abounds.

BY GINA KOLATA
The New York Times, May 3, 2011

A new study found that low-salt diets increase the risk of death from heart attacks and strokes and do not prevent high blood pressure, *but the research's limitations mean the debate over the effects of salt in the* diet *is far from over.*

Dr. Peter Briss, a medical director at the centers, said that the study was small; *that its subjects were relatively young, with an average age of 40 at the start; and that with few cardiovascular events, it was hard to draw conclusions. And the study, Dr. Briss and others say, flies in the face of a body of evidence indicating that higher sodium consumption can increase the risk of cardiovascular disease.*

The study is published in the May 4 issue of The Journal of the American Medical Association. It involved only those without high blood pressure at the start, was observational, considered at best suggestive and not conclusive. It included 3,681 middle-aged Europeans who did not have high blood pressure or cardio-vascular disease and followed them for an average of 7.9 years.

The investigators found that the less salt people ate, the more likely they were to die of heart disease . . . "If the goal is to prevent hypertension" with lower sodium consumption, said the lead author, Dr. Jan A. Staessen, . . . "this study shows it does not work."

One problem with the salt debates, Dr. Alderman said, is that all the studies are inadequate. Either they are short-term intervention studies in which people are given huge amounts of salt and then deprived of salt to see effects on blood pressure or they are studies, like this one, that observe populations and ask if those who happen to consume less salt are healthier.

"Observational studies tell you what people will experience if they select

a diet," Dr. Alderman said. "They do not tell you what will happen if you change peoples' sodium intake. What is needed . . . is a large study in which people are randomly assigned to follow a low-sodium diet or not and followed for years to see if eating less salt improves health and reduces the death rate from cardiovascular disease."

"This is one of those really interesting situations," said Dr. Lawrence Appel, ... "You can say, 'O.K., let's dismiss the observational studies because they have all these problems.' " But, he said, despite the virtues of a randomized controlled clinical trial, such a study "will never ever be done." It would be impossible to keep people on a low-sodium diet for years with so much sodium added to prepared foods.

This story in the *New York Times* is reporting on the controversy that ensued after a research study on low salt diets was published.

Read what is being said about the study's research design. The study used an observational design (non experimental). Some critics say a randomized controlled trial (experimental study) was needed here.

Can you draw a cause and effect relationship if a non-experimental approach is used?

Can you say that a low salt diet causes heart attacks and strokes as a result of the findings of this study?

Is it possible to do an experimental study such as the one suggested by Dr. Alderman (e.g., a "large study in which people are randomly assigned to follow a low-sodium diet or not and followed for years to see if eating less salt improves health and reduces the death rate from cardiovascular disease")?

Will the results of this study change the way nurses intervene with patients on a low salt diet?

What would you say to a relative on a low salt diet that read about this study and wanted to quit his diet?

> **Consider This . . .**
>
> Would you use an experimental or a non-experimental design to answer the research
> question that you identified for your clinical problem? Hint: Ask yourself whether you are
> interested in finding a cause and effect relationship.

Check out Box 5-4 again. The first hypothesis in Example 2 represents a non-experimental design. The independent variable is the presence or absence of IBS. This variable cannot be manipulated (because the researcher cannot induce IBS in participants). Instead, the researchers found participants who were already diagnosed with IBS or who had no IBS and compared stress and distress levels in the two groups. Now look at the first hypothesis in Example 1. This clearly represents an experimental design. The researcher is manipulating the independent variable. One group of abused women is given a specified case management intervention and the other group is only given an information card. Here the researcher is testing to see whether the case management intervention is effective in getting the women to use safety behaviors. We will discuss research designs in greater detail and explore specific experimental and non-experimental design types in Chapter 6.

Identify the Population and Sample

Once the research design has been established, the researcher must decide where the study will take place and who will participate in the study. The **setting** refers to the physical location for and the conditions under which the study will take place. For example, in the study that studied women with and without IBS, the setting was the local community. In the study that worked with abused women, two public health clinics served as the setting.

POPULATION. The participants that the researcher wants to study are known as a **population**. These participants possess certain common characteristics that identify them as a part of the population. Check out Box 5-3 again. In Example 1, the population is adolescents with diabetes. In Example 2, the population is people with diabetes who are found in an acute care setting. Participants need not be human. Animals, viral colonies, DNA strands, or medical records might serve as populations of interest. A **sample** is a smaller piece of the population of interest, as shown in Figure 5-3. Populations are usually large, so a part of the population is selected to make executing the study more possible.

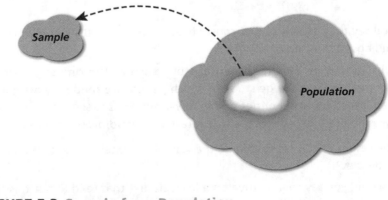

■ **FIGURE 5-3 Sample from Population**
(Adapted from Langford 2001)
A smaller portion is drawn out of the population.

This process of selecting a subset of the population is known as **sampling.** The procedures used in this sampling process are designed to make the sample characteristics match the population characteristics as closely as possible. When sample characteristics reflect the characteristics of the population, the sample is said to be representative. This is important because a representative sample allows the application of the study findings back to the population. For example, if the abused women in the intimate partner violence study were shown to use more safety behaviors after receiving the case management intervention, it is helpful if that finding can be applied to all women abused by an intimate partner. The ability to apply study results from the sample to the population is known as **generalizability**. The type of sampling process chosen determines whether study results can be generalized from the sample to the population.

There are two major ways to classify sampling methods: 1) probability and 2) non-probability. **Probability samples** ensure that samples are mathematically representative of the population. That means that each element (person, animal, or object) in the population has an equal and independent chance of being in the sample. When researchers choose probability sampling techniques, they ensure that the results of the study can be generalized to the population. Subjects in **non-probability samples** are not chosen at random. Thus there is no way to truly determine whether or not they are representative of the population. This means that when a study chooses to use a non-probability sampling technique, the findings cannot be generalized to the population with any confidence.

Consider This . . .

How might the selection of a non-probability sample affect the trust you would place in the final results?

PROBABILITY SAMPLING. Probability sampling is also called random sampling because of the random process involved in selecting participants. This precise sampling process means that every participant in a defined population has an equal chance of being selected for the sample. There are four types of probability sampling techniques: 1) simple random sampling, 2) stratified random sampling, 3) cluster or multistage sampling, and 4) systematic random sampling.

Simple random sampling is the most common form of random sampling. Here a list of the population is obtained and numbered and numbers are then selected using a technique such as a table of random numbers or a lottery. There is even computerized random number generator software available to make this a simpler process. A stratified random sample is much the same except the population list is subdivided into smaller groups by some trait or characteristic such as race or gender before the selection process. Participants are then drawn from each of the newly formed groupings. In cluster sampling, there is a successive random sampling of various population clusters. This cluster approach starts by randomly selecting large groups such as primary care clinics. They then take the selected clinics and randomly choose smaller clusters such as individual patients from those clinics. A systematic sample involves the selection of every k^{th} participant from a randomized list, such as every 50th nurse on a random list of registered nurses in the state of Texas. The key here is that the names on the list must be randomly ordered (alphabetical lists or lists sorted by zip code, for instance, would not be considered random).

NON-PROBABILITY SAMPLING. There are also four non-probability sampling techniques: 1) convenience sampling, 2) quota sampling, 3) purposive sampling, and 4) systematic sampling. Convenience sampling, the most common form of sampling, selects the most conveniently available participants, such as the first 50 people admitted to a hospital emergency center with a laceration. Quota sampling looks somewhat like stratified random sampling. Participants are drawn from certain predefined groups such as males and females. However, there is no random process at work here. If researchers want 25 males and 25 females in the ER laceration study, they simply choose the first 25 males and the first 25 females. In purposive sampling the participants are hand selected by the researchers based on some set of criteria. For example, researchers might want to choose experts on the topic that they are researching. Non-probability systematic sampling uses the same selection procedures as random systematic sampling with one important difference: the population list is not randomly ordered. For example the list might be alphabetized.

When reading research articles, be aware that researchers do not always clearly label the type of sampling technique they used, particularly when it was a convenience technique. However, you can often figure out the technique by reading the description. Box 5-5 shows some non-probability sample descriptions.

BOX 5-5 Non-Probability Sampling Examples

Convenience: In the study of diabetic adolescents and summer camp (Cheung et al. 2006), participants were conveniently selected as indicated by the following: "Participants were adolescents with diabetes who were listed in a database available from the DSSCV. The first 100 participants from the directory were chosen to participate" (p. 55).

Convenience: Another convenience sampling example is found in the rural exercise program study (Bennett et al. 2008). "Eligible participants (from four rural health clinics) were underactive rural adults aged 25 years and older who were willing to try to increase their physical activity . . . Participants were excluded only if they had a medical condition that contraindicated participation in moderate-intensity exercise for 6 months or if they had no telephone . . . If the patient agreed to be contacted, study staff telephoned to describe the study and enroll the participant" (p. 25).

Quota: A description of a quota sampling technique is much more directly identified in a study examining participants in clinical trials (Rabin and Tabak 2006) with the statement that "The study design is quasi-experimental, using a convenience quota sample" (p. 974).

Purposive: A study (Gilje, Klose, and Birger 2007) of clinical competencies in undergraduate psychiatric mental health nursing used "A purposive sample of 18 nurses with (extensive) experience in psychiatric care and nursing education completed a 198-item survey . . ." (p. 522)

Use of random selection techniques tend to be more clearly identified. See Box 5-6 for examples of probability samples.

GENERALIZABILITY. The ability to generalize the results becomes very important to note when you read and apply research studies to your practice. Generalizability allows you to apply the study results to your situation. So, if a probability sample of patients possesses characteristics similar to patients under your care, you can confidently apply the study findings to your patients. If a non-probability sample was used, you have no way to know with any confidence whether the findings are applicable to your patients.

BOX 5-6 Probability Samples

Simple random: In a study by Manojilovich (2005) that examined predictors of professional nursing practice: "The sample consisted of 500 nurses randomly selected from a list of 1,509 names provided by the Michigan Nurses Association" (p. 43).

Stratified Random: A study by Lazenblatt and Freeman (2006) describes a stratified random sample. "A stratified sampling frame was designed to select participants randomly from the list of all CNs, GDPs and GMPs in NI using a table of random numbers. Names of GMPs and GDPs were obtained from the NI Council for Postgraduate Medical and Dental Education and Central Services Agency (Central Service Agency 2003a,b, Office for National Statistics 2002). CNs were accessed via Health and Social Services Trusts and the Community Health Visitors Association. The minimum sample size to satisfy requirements was estimated to be 146 for each category of professional" (p. 229).

Cluster Sample: A study by Leonhardt et al. (2008) used a multisite cluster approach and described it right in the study title. "TTM-based motivational counselling does not increase physical activity of low back pain patients in a primary care setting—A cluster-randomized controlled trial" (p. 50).

If probability samples allow researchers to generalize their findings to a larger population then why would most researchers choose non-probability techniques? It usually has something to do with expense, resources, or time. Non-probability techniques are generally less expensive, require less time, and use fewer resources than random sampling. Think about compiling and numbering a list of 5,000 or 10,000 elements in a population. Even if such lists are computerized, this could be a daunting and time consuming task.

The size of the sample is also important in ensuring that it is truly representative. Generally, the larger the sample, the more representative it is of the population. When you read a research study, check the sample size. If a sample is small (under 30) and a non-probability technique was used, consider the study results with caution. Refer back to the *Research in the News* box. One of the criticisms was that the sample of nearly 4,000 was too small. Would you consider the sample to be too small?

Select Instruments for Data Collection

Once researchers choose the sample and sampling technique, they must develop a plan and locate instruments to collect data on the identified variables in the study. **Instruments** are simply devices or techniques that are used to gather the data. For quantitative research, the data must be collected in such a way that it can be turned into a numerical score. This score represents a measurement of the variable and will be used in statistical analysis in Phase 4.

Data are measurable bits of information and can be generally classified as physiological, behavioral, or psychological in nature. Physiological measures usually require specialized biophysical devices that are commonly used in health care and in health care research. In fact, we use many of these instruments in our daily clinical practice. Common examples include thermometers to measure body temperature, sphygmomanometers to measure blood pressure, glucometers to measure blood sugar, and pulse oximeters to measure oxygen saturation. We also use more complex instruments such as x-rays, EKGs and EEGs, CT scans, and MRIs to measure physiologic variables. Laboratory analysis can be used to measure the properties of blood, urine, and assorted body tissues.

When studying a behavioral variable, data is best collected through structured observation of the participants. Researchers might use a checklist to note the frequency of occurrence of the behavior, a rating scale to note the intensity of the behavior, or a categorized list to classify the behavior. For example, handwashing might be observed for frequency of occurrence and for technique used (e.g. time taken, surfaces washed, use of soap). Intake and output of fluid in an ICU might be observed and recorded on a flow sheet. Respirations might be observed by counting the number of rise and falls of the patient's chest during a 1-minute interval.

If the researcher wants to assess knowledge, feelings, attitudes, or beliefs, then he or she would use psychological measures to collect data. Since these variables cannot be directly observed, they must be measured by asking the participant about them. This is known as a self-report. Researchers typically use questionnaires or interviews to collect this type of data. Regardless of format, these questionnaires and interviews are highly structured in order to produce a numerical score. Questionnaires are easy to administer, inexpensive, and can be mailed or offered over the Internet to a large, widely dispersed sample. A structured interview is much like giving a scale or questionnaire in oral form. The advantage of an interview is the ability to clarify responses and to ensure that all the items are completed. The major disadvantages are the increased time and expense of the process and the inability to easily access large or dispersed populations.

You have used many self-report measures, whether you realize it or not. When you take an exam, it serves as a self-report measure of your knowledge. When a marketer stops you in the supermarket and asks you what brand of tuna you buy, your answer is a self-report of your buying habits. When a nurse asks you to rate your pain on a scale of 1 to 10, your reply is a self-report. Self-report can be as simple and direct as answering the question "How do you feel today?" It can also be as complex as filling out a 50-item scale that asks you to rate how you feel on a number of parameters using a 5-point scale (known as a Likert scale) from always to never. Self-report questionnaires are the most widely used form of data collection in nursing research.

Before making the final selection of an instrument, researchers must address the critical issue of whether it is reliable and valid. A reliable instrument measures the variable dependably, consistently, and accurately. A valid instrument measures what it is designed to measure.

RELIABILITY. **Reliability** examines the dependability of an instrument. There are three major types of reliability: 1) internal consistency, 2) stability, and 3) equivalence. Internal consistency is usually calculated for self-report instruments such as multi-item Likert scales. The internal consistency measure determines whether the items of a particular scale all measure the same trait. It is reported as a correlation statistic such as a Cronbach's alpha or Kuder-Richardson. Values are displayed as r values and range from 0 to 1. The closer the value gets to 1, the more reliable the instrument (.7 or above is considered acceptable, and .8 or above is desirable).

Stability is assessed by determining whether an instrument gets similar results when administered on different occasions over time. The instrument is administered two times and the two scores are correlated. The r values will range from 0 to 1 and values above .70 are deemed acceptable.

Equivalence may be assessed on two different occasions. It may be used to determine whether two different forms of an instrument have a similar score (also called parallel forms). Equivalence for parallel forms is reported as a correlation coefficient (r of .70 is adequate, .80 or above is desirable). Equivalence may also be used to determine whether two different raters or observers agree on their scoring. This is also called interrater reliability. Interrater reliability is reported as a correlation coefficient (an r of .7 or above is acceptable) or as a Cohen's kappa (k of .6 or above is acceptable).

VALIDITY. **Validity** is the extent to which an instrument measures what it says it measures. An instrument can have 1) content validity, 2) criterion validity, or 3) construct validity.

Content validity is assessed by using a logical evaluation of whether the instrument adequately reflects the universe of content for a particular concept. A blueprint may have been used to construct the instrument or a panel of judges may have been asked to evaluate the instrument. This is considered a fairly weak form of validity.

Consider This ...

If a research study used an instrument that was not reliable or valid, what impact would that have on your decision to use the results of that study?

Researchers use statistical measures to assess criterion validity. They correlate instrument scores to scores on measures of some external criteria. If the scores correlate highly the instrument is deemed as valid. This is a stronger form of validity than content validity, but requires the use of an external measure that is known to be reliable. The question is, why use a second instrument that must be validated by already established criteria? Why not just use the established criteria? It may be that the external criteria are difficult or expensive to measure. For example, you might want to measure percentage of body fat. You could use a hydrostatic measure, which is proven and reliable. However, this requires submerging the person in a large tank of water and measuring the amount of water that is displaced by the submerged body. Such tank measures are usually found in specialized laboratories. If a researcher could measure skin folds using skin calipers and obtain a similar measure of body fat, it would be much less expensive, less time consuming, and require minimal equipment. So a high correlation of the two measures could test the validity of the skin caliper method.

Construct validity is assessed using a combination of logical and statistical measures. It looks for the underlying meaning of the construct being measured. Construct validity uses statistical techniques such as the multitrait-multimethod matrix method (MTMM) or factor analysis to provide statistical evidence that underlying theoretical constructs are being measured. This is considered the strongest form of validity.

As you read a research article you should look for evidence that the researchers used reliable and valid instruments to measure the variables in the study. You should expect to see information about the reliability and validity of the instruments used. This allows you to make judgements about the quality of the data collected. If the data are suspect then the study results are suspect. Reliability and validity for biophysical measures are often reported by describing the procedure for data collection, and the type or calibration of equipment. Psychological scales that have been tested extensively for reliability and validity are considered to be standardized, and the researcher may not address reliability and validity issues. In these instances, the onus is on the reader to recognize that the instrument being used is standardized. The research article should also contain a brief description of the instrument(s) used. Box 5-7 gives examples of studies using various types of instruments and reporting methods for reliability and validity.

In Example 1, the dependent variable was stress response and it was measured using four biomarkers (biophysical). Reliability and validity is addressed by describing the collection procedure and noting the labs that performed the tests. In Example 2, the dependent variable was coping and was measured using a self-report scale. The researchers discussed reliability and validity, implying that the instrument was standardized. They also reported an internal consistency measure (called the Cronbach alpha) for the study sample. In Example 3, the study examined a number of dependent variables including threats of violence and physical assaults. These variables were measured using a self-report pen-and-paper questionnaire. Internal consistency was reported for past studies as

---

BOX 5-7 Study Examples of Instruments and Instrument Quality

Example 1: From the Chlan et al. (2007) study: "Influence of music on the stress response in patients receiving mechanical ventilatory support"

"Blood samples were obtained from the central venous catheter . . . *Corticotropin and Cortisol Assays.* Approximately 5 mL of blood was placed in a siliconized, lavender glass tube. Plasma level of corticotropin was assayed with direct radioimmunoassay; plasma level of cortisol was measured with a radioimmunoassay kit (ICN Biochemical, Costa Mesa, Calif). *Epinephrine and Norepinephrine Assays.* Approximately 7 mL of blood was placed in a heparinized glass collection tube. Epinephrine and norepinephrine were assayed by using high-performance liquid chromatography with electrochemical detection; the assay was performed by a diagnostic laboratory (ARUP Laboratories, Salt Lake City, Utah)" (p. 142).

Example 2: From the Jalowiec et al. (2007) study: "Predictors of Perceived Coping Effectiveness in Patients Awaiting a Heart Transplant"

"The 1987 revised version of the Jalowiec Coping Scale (JCS) was used to assess coping behavior . . . (JCS) measures the use and the perceived effectiveness of 60 cognitive and behavioral coping strategies on 0 to 3 rating scales . . . The JCS has been used internationally in numerous studies with many different populations and age groups since the first version in 1977 . . . The JCS has good reliability and validity from previous studies . . . Alpha reliability for the total effectiveness score from the present sample was .92 . . ." (p. 262).

Example 3: From the McFarlane et al. (2006) study: "Secondary prevention of intimate partner violence: A randomized controlled trial"

"The Severity of Violence Against Women Scale (SVAWS) is a 46-item instrument designed to measure threats of physical violence (19 items) and physical assault (27 items) (Marshall 1992). Examples of behaviors that represent physical violence are kicking, choking, beating up, and forced sex. For each item, the woman responds using a 4-point scale to indicate how often the behavior occurred (0 = never, 1 = once, 2 = 2-3 times, 3 = 4 or more times). The possible range of scores was 0 to 57 for the threats of abuse and 0 to 81 for physical assault. Internal consistency reliability estimates for abused women have ranged from .89 to .91 for threats of abuse and .91 to .94 for assault (Gist et al., 2001; Wiist & McFarlane, 1998a, 1998b). For the present study, reliability, as measured by Cronbach's alpha, was .92 for both threats of abuse and physical assault" (p. 4).

well as the current study. Validity was not addressed. However, it is evident that this tool has been used in previous studies.

Phase 3: Implement the Design

The researcher is now ready to conduct the study using the framework and design developed in the first two phases. This is an exciting time in the process for most researchers as the study begins to take full shape. There are three steps in this phase. Researchers must first address ethical considerations that might occur during data collection. Then they recruit study participants and collect the data.

Address Ethical Considerations

As you learned in Chapter 4, any participant in a research study has certain basic rights. First and foremost, they have the right to be free from harm and to be treated with respect. Researchers are obligated to protect subjects from potential discomfort or harm that might occur as a result of participating in the research study and must treat participants sensitively and courteously. Participants have a right to privacy. Researchers must put procedures into place that ensure that participant identity is protected and that participant results are confidential. Finally, participants have the right to know what to expect and to freely choose to be a part of the study. Researchers must obtain informed consent from potential participants and must allow the person to freely decide if they wish participate. The informed consent must spell out the possible risks and benefits associated with the study.

How do we ensure that researchers provide these basic rights for their study participants? Prior to conducting a research study, researchers must receive approval from the appropriate institutional review boards (IRBs). If you recall from the discussion in Chapter 4, IRBs are review groups that have been formed by universities, hospitals, or other health care institutions and are charged with the responsibility of ensuring that individuals who conduct research in their institutions adhere to certain ethical standards.

> **Consider This . . .**
>
> Do you think review by one committee is enough to protect participants in a research study? Why or why not? What if the review board is a hospital that stands to benefit if grant monies are attached to the proposed study?

The first step in this phase is to obtain IRB approval. The researcher submits a written proposal of the research study to the appropriate IRB and addresses participant rights and plans to protect these rights. The IRB reviews the proposal using specified U.S. Department of Health and Human Services (USDHHS) guidelines and awards or denies authorization for the conduct of the study. If more than one institution is involved in the study, the researcher must seek approval from the IRB in each institution. This process is known as dual review. When authorization is granted by all participating institutions, the researcher can then start the process of recruiting subjects for data collection.

Recruit Participants

The first step in recruiting is to find potential participants. The researcher has already spelled out the criteria for inclusion in the sample and has designated where the data will be collected in the first step of Phase 2. At this point the researcher often uses a screening form at the data collection site to quickly determine who is eligible for the study. Once eligible individuals have been identified, the researcher must persuade them to join the study. Effective recruitment strategies involve a courteous and sensitive face-to-face recruitment technique that carefully delineates the benefits of participation. Researchers should also strive to make participation as easy and convenient as possible. Some researchers have found that the use of incentives such as gifts or money is helpful.

Consider This ...

What are some issues or ethical dilemmas that might arise if participants are offered money to participate in a study?

Once an individual has agreed to participate, the researcher obtains informed consent stating that the participant has been briefed on the study and is willing to participate. A typical consent form usually contains a brief statement of the study purpose, a description of study procedures, a list of potential risks and benefits, assurance of confidentiality, and assurance that participation is voluntary and that the participant may withdraw without penalty. The participant receives a copy of the signed consent form with contact information for the researcher and an offer to answer any questions about the study.

Some studies do not require written informed consent. When written questionnaires are used, return of the questionnaire is frequently used to imply consent. Informed consent might unwittingly alter study results in certain observational studies, so IRBs may also allow researchers to conduct certain observations without obtaining informed consent so long as the researcher produces sufficient evidence that identifying information about participants will be kept confidential.

Collect Data

Once researchers obtain permission from the appropriate IRBs and recruit their subjects they can proceed with data collection. At this point, the researchers put the design into action and carry out the prescribed procedures for the study in the appropriate research setting. They conduct treatments, administer instruments, and generate and record data. After the data are collected, the researcher organizes that data into an appropriate form for analysis and Phase 3 is brought to a close.

As you read published research you will see some description of this phase. You should expect some mention of IRB approval and of informed consent as well as a cursory description of data collection. Box 5-8 provides some examples of Phase 3 study descriptions. Note that in Example 1, the study directly states that IRB approval and informed consent were obtained and a description of the data collection procedure is provided. In Example 2, the study states that IRB approval and informed consent were obtained and a glimpse of recruitment and data collection procedures is given, including the use of an incentive. Finally, in Example 3, the study provides a broader explanation of Phase 3 activities. In addition to a statement of IRB approval and informed consent, recruitment procedures are described in fair detail including nurse training to enhance identification and recruitment of potential participants. The informed consent process was detailed, the data collection process was described, and there was a description of the use of incentives.

> ## BOX 5-8 Research Study Examples of Phase 3 Descriptions
>
> ### Example 1: From the Chlan et al. (2007) study "Influence of music on the stress response in patients receiving mechanical ventilatory support"
>
> "A convenience sample was recruited from an 11-bed medical intensive care unit (ICU) in a university-affiliated medical center in the urban Midwest after approval was received from the university's institutional review board . . . Subjects provided their own informed consent . . . Beginning at 5:40 AM, blood samples were obtained from the central venous catheter at 4 intervals: baseline, 15 minutes after baseline, 30 minutes after baseline, and 60 minutes after baseline. Specimens were transferred to their respective collection tubes and immediately placed on ice" (p. 142).
>
> ### Example 2: From the Jalowiec et al. (2007) study "Predictors of Perceived Coping Effectiveness in Patients Awaiting a Heart Transplant"
>
> "This research was approved by the Institutional Review Board at both sites [Loyola University of Chicago and the University of Alabama at Birmingham]. Data were collected by patient completion of a booklet of questionnaires on multiple factors impacting on quality of life and by retrieval of chart data by RN research assistants. Patients were approached onsite at the clinic or hospital to see if they wanted to participate in the study. After receiving an explanation of the study requirements and reviewing the booklet, patients gave written consent to participate. Patients returned the completed booklet by mail if they were not hospitalized at study entry . . . Patients were paid $10 for each booklet completed" (p. 261).
>
> ### Example 3: From the McFarlane et al. (2006) study "Secondary prevention of intimate partner violence: A randomized controlled trial"
>
> "Prior to study implementation . . . a training program [for registered nurses] included didactic sessions and activities to aid the nurses in referring abused women to appropriate community services. For the woman who was positive for abuse . . . the research nurses gave an explanation of the study purpose, protocol, instruments, administration time, and follow-up schedule. Following an informed consent procedure completed by the nurse, the nurse verbally administered the interview questionnaire, then provided the designated intervention . . . Instruments were available in English and Spanish and were administered in a private room without the partner or other individuals being present . . . To compensate the participants for their time, each woman was offered a $20 stipend for the first interview, $20 for the 6-month interview, $30 for the 12-month interview, $30 for the 18-month interview, and $40 for the 24-month interview. Data collection began after institutional review board and clinic approvals were obtained" (pp. 2–3).

Phase 4: Analyze and Interpret the Data

Researchers must analyze and interpret the data they collect. Statistical analysis is the hallmark of a quantitative study and one of the major distinctions between quantitative and qualitative research. The statistical analysis accomplishes two major tasks: It provides a description of the sample in the study and answers the research questions or hypotheses which were proposed in Phase 1. Once the data has been statistically analyzed and described, the results are translated into narrative form.

Describe the Sample

When analyzing the participants in a study, the researcher describes what the sample looks like on a number of characteristics such as age, gender, race, and diagnosis. These characteristics are selected by the researcher as being relevant to that particular group of participants. Statistics are used to aid in this description. These **descriptive statistics** examine the data on these selected characteristics in standard ways that make the description concise and easier to picture. There are three common ways to describe data using statistics: 1) frequencies, 2) measures of central tendency, and 3) measures of spread.

FREQUENCIES. Frequencies are a very basic way to describe the data. The researcher simply counts the number of times a value occurs for a certain characteristic. For example, if gender were the characteristic that the researcher wanted to describe, he/she would look at the data and count the number of males and females in the sample. Those frequencies can then be converted to percentages. Table 5-1 gives you an example of frequencies and percentages that were gathered on gender, ethnicity, and identified health problems in a sample of 34 overweight and obese adolescents. This gives the researcher and the reader a concise picture about the participants in the study. When viewing Table 5-1, you can instantly envision the number and percentage of males and females in this sample.

Frequencies work well when we are reporting on characteristics that have a manageable number of categories like gender or ethnicity. However, suppose the characteristic of interest was age or height or weight? Reporting frequencies of counts for these

▶ **Table 5-1   Gender, Race, and Health Problem Frequencies for Adolescent Sample**

Variable	Frequency	Percent
Gender		
Male	13	38.2
Female	21	61.8
Ethnicity		
Caucasian	5	14.7
African American	6	17.6
Hispanic	20	58.9
Other	3	8.8
Health Problems		
HTN	3	8.8
High Cholesterol	3	8.8
Acanthosis	17	50.0
2 or more problems	2	5.9
No Problems	9	26.5
N = 34		

characteristics could make for a very long table that isn't very helpful. So, when researchers use frequencies for these variables, they group several values together and report frequencies for a group of values. Let's look at the age and body mass index (BMI) for our adolescent sample in Table 5-2.

▶ Table 5-2 Age and Weight Frequencies for Adolescent Sample		
Variable	**Frequency**	**Percent**
Age		
11-13	9	26.5
14-16	14	41.1
17-19	11	32.4
BMI		
25-29.9	7	20.6
30-39.9	15	44.1
40 and over	12	35.3
N=34		

Data that produces numbers that can be ordered from low to high and have an infinite number of values in a defined range are called continuous data. Age and BMI are good examples. Researchers can represent continuous data as a frequency distribution and plot them on a graph. Figure 5-4 plots the data from Table 5-2.

You will seldom see graphs in a research article. However, frequency distributions serve another purpose. They allow the researcher to describe what are called measures of central tendency and measures of spread for that frequency distribution.

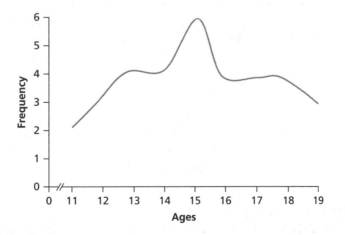

■ **FIGURE 5-4** Example of a Frequency Distribution
Plotting the data as a graph makes it even easier to see the frequency distribution (note the spike at age 15).

MEASURES OF CENTRAL TENDENCY. Measures of central tendency describe how data for a particular characteristic tend to cluster together in a distribution. There are three measures of central tendency. You are probably most familiar with the measure of central tendency known as the mean (x). The mean is the average of all the values for a particular characteristic. For example, the mean age in the adolescent sample is 15.21. Calculating a mean is an easy procedure. You just add up all the scores and divide by the number of scores you added together.

The other two measures of central tendency are the mode, which is the numerical value that occurs most often for a particular characteristic, and the median, which is the middle value in a frequency distribution. If we look at the frequency distribution for age in Figure 5-3, then age 15 would be the mode. It is easy to find the median when there are an odd number of values in the sample: just pick the value in the middle. When the sample values are even, as are the ages in the adolescent sample, find the two middle scores and average them. So for age of the adolescents, we would take the 16th and the 17th values and average them. In this case, both the 16th and 17th values are age 15, so our median is 15. Note how the mean, median, and mode are very similar for the sample distribution.

MEASURES OF DISPERSION. Measures of dispersion tell us that values tend to spread out on the frequency distribution. There are also three measures of dispersion. The easiest measure of dispersion is called a range. To find the range, simply subtract the lowest value from the highest value. In our example of adolescent age, we would subtract 11 from 19 and our range would be 8. The other two measures are the variance and the standard deviation, which are mathematically derived numbers. The variance (V) is the average area of spread under the frequency distribution curve and the standard deviation (SD) is the average distance of spread in a frequency distribution. The key things to remember are that both measures tell us how much the scores are spread out from the mean on average, and the larger the values, the greater the spread. The variance for age in the adolescent sample was 5.34 and the standard deviation was 2.31.

All of these descriptive statistics allow the researcher to describe the sample in a concise and precise manner. When you read a research study, the sample description can help you to determine whether the sample characteristics are similar to or different from the groups to which you want to apply the results of the study. Box 5-9 illustrates two sample descriptions. The first is in the form of a table found in an article by Cheung et al. (2006). The second is a narrative description found in an article by Hertig et al. (2007). If you were reading the studies in Box 5-9, you could compare the variables described in the study with the group of individuals you are interested in to see whether they are similar. If they are similar, you as a reader can feel more confident in applying the results of the study to the individuals you work with. For example, suppose you work with adolescents, some of whom are diabetic, and you want to know whether a referral to a summer camp would help with your patients' quality of life. The descriptive statistics let you compare the adolescents in the study with the adolescents that you work with.

Present the Findings

Having described the sample, the researcher can now explore the data collected on the research problem. Researchers use statistics that allow them to find the answers to the research question they posed or to assess whether their data prove their hypotheses. These answers are what the researcher designed the study for. The statistics used to find

BOX 5-9 Example of a Sample Description

Example 1: Table

The table (Cheung et al. 2006) reveals frequencies and percentages for the study variables: attendance, number of camps, age, and gender.

Table I.   Demographic Information ($n = 39$)

	n	%
Attendance in diabetes camp		
Yes	29	74
Number of camps		
1–3	25	64
>3	4	10
None	10	26
Age		
13–15 years	28	72
16–17 years	11	28
Gender		
Female	23	59
Male	16	41

Note. Not all per percentages equal 100% because of rounding

Example 2: Narrative

The narrative below describes the variables age, ethnicity, partnered status, occupation, education, and income from the Hertig et al. (2007) study. Here the description is more general. It primarily informs the reader that the IBS and comparison group were alike on these variables.

"On average, the participants were 32 years of age and predominantly Caucasian (85%), and 49% were married or partnered. There were no significant differences in age, ethnicity, partnered status, occupation, education, and income between women with IBS and women in the comparison group. Similarly, there were no differences in demographic characteristics across IBS bowel pattern subgroups. Of the total sample, over half of the women ($n = 159$) had completed college, a third ($n = 88$) held professional managerial positions, and 43 were students" (p. 402).

these answers are often complex and may be beyond your understanding at this point in your education. Fortunately for you, however, the researcher will interpret the statistical results for you, so do not panic when you see the numbers and tables of numbers. Instead search for the answers to the research questions or the hypotheses, which is often reported in the Discussion section. These are known as the study **findings** and are simply the results of the statistical analysis that was done on the data. You really only need only one key piece of information: *Were the findings significant or not?* For example, if the treatment worked, then the study will report a significant difference between the control group and the treatment group. If two variables were related to one another, the study will report a significant relationship. Check out Box 5-10 for examples of findings. You will see that you can locate and understand the answers to the questions or hypotheses posed by the researchers.

Interpret the Findings

Once the answers have been discovered to the questions/hypotheses posed, the researcher must determine how those answers fit into the larger picture. This means determining how the findings fit into the existing research that was discovered during the literature review process. If the findings were what the researcher expected, then interpretation is relatively easy. Since the researcher based the research questions or hypotheses on a theoretical frame of reference, expected findings lend support to the theoretical approach chosen and add support to or extend the findings that were already available in the literature. If the findings were unexpected, then the researcher must try to explain what why. Explanations may range from a reexamination of the theoretical underpinnings of the study to searching for limitations in the research design or the sample size.

BOX 5-10 Examples of Study Findings

Example 1: Answering a research question

Remember the study question asked by Cheung et al. (2006): "Is QOL in adolescents with diabetes who attend diabetes camp higher than the QOL in adolescents with diabetes who have never attended diabetes camp?" The answer is reported below.

"Independent sample *t* tests comparing respondents from the AC [camp] and NC [no camp] groups were used. . . . Results showed no statistically significant differences for these three subcategories [of the Diabetes Quality of life scale]" (p. 56) and . . . "The findings indicated no significant difference in QOL among adolescents who attend diabetes camp and those who did not" (p. 57).

Example 2: Answering a research hypothesis

Hertig et al. (2008) tested two hypotheses: 1. "Women with IBS will report higher levels of stress and psychological distress compared with women without IBS." and 2. "Intensity of stress will be associated with severity of abdominal discomfort symptoms and bowel pattern symptoms" (p. 400). Here are the reported answers for these two hypotheses.

"Women with IBS report significantly more stress and greater psychological distress as compared with women in the comparison group. . . . Second, across women, stress is associated significantly with severity of abdominal discomfort symptoms but not bowel pattern symptoms. The strongest associations, however, are seen between stress and psychological distress" (pp. 403–404).

> ### BOX 5-11   Study Examples of Interpreting the Findings
>
> **Example 1: Unexpected results—(Cheung et al. 2006)**
>
> "The small sample size was a major limitation of this study. More time and follow-up reminders may have resulted in a larger number of participants. Ten (10%) of the questionnaires were returned as undeliverable. . . . This study could have a type II error, a false retention of the null hypothesis. Because of the cost of mailing, the researcher was unable to send questionnaire packets to every participant listed in the DSSCV directory. The study may have yielded more statistically significant results if more packets had been distributed, thus increasing the number of packets returned" (p. 57).
>
> **Example 2: Expected results—(Hertig et al. 2007)**
>
> "Abdominal pain, bloating, and intestinal gas are correlated more strongly with stress than are the bowel pattern symptoms constipation and diarrhea. Abdominal pain in particular is shown to have the greatest impact on quality of life indicators in women with IBS (Cain et al., 2006; Lembo et al., 1999)" (p. 405) and . . . "Data from this group support the influence of stress and corticotropin releasing hormone in the regulation of intestinal epithelial and immune function via mast cell activation (Santos, Guilarte, Alonso, & Malagelada, 2005)" (p. 405).

In Box 5-11, you will find the interpretations from the findings that were illustrated and discussed in Box 5-10. In Example 1, the findings were unexpected. Note that the researcher addresses this issue by looking at sample size and recruitment issues. In Example 2, the study results were expected. Note that in this case, the researchers place their results in context of the literature.

Phase 5: Use the Results

Phase 4 transitions nicely into Phase 5. The researcher begins this phase by making recommendations for further research and by suggesting possible implications of the results for use in professional practice. An **implication** is an inference drawn about the study results which determines what the study means in terms of practice and research. In this phase, then, the researcher examines the contributions that the study makes to the practice of nursing and offers suggestions for future research. This leads to the final responsibility of the researcher and the first step in this phase, which is to disseminate the findings.

Disseminate the Findings

The researchers' job is not complete until the results are shared with a wider audience of nurses and other health care professionals. This is known as **dissemination**. This is usually accomplished in two major ways. The results could be presented in oral or written form at a professional conference, or the results could be published in a professional journal. Presentations allow the results to be broadcast in a rapid and timely manner and can stimulate dialog among professionals who share similar interests. Published articles may not reach the audience until 1 to 2 years after the study is completed. However, given the ready access to electronic forms, journals have the advantage of a worldwide distribution. Most researchers opt for both options.

Use the Findings in Nursing Practice

The final step is a key one in the process and belongs to you as a practicing nurse. The research consumer (you) must now take the disseminated results and apply them in professional practice.

> **Consider This . . .**
>
> What would you say to persuade a colleague who did not see the value of reading nursing research literature that reading research could improve the practice of nursing?

It is the translation of research into practice that ensures building one's practice on a foundation of the best available scientific evidence. You have a professional obligation to develop and improve your nursing practice using the most currently available research-generated knowledge. As you and other health care professionals use the research findings, new problems will surface and present themselves for research. The primary aim of this book is to provide you with the necessary tools to read and apply research findings to improve and keep your practice current. In doing so you provide researchers with new problems for research and the cycle is continued. Research and practice rely on one another to ensure the best care possible.

SUMMARY

In this chapter, you scrutinized the 5 phases of the quantitative research process in greater detail, examining the steps that comprise each phase. You reviewed examples of key concepts from actual nursing research studies. Here is a summary of the key points in this chapter.

- **Quantitative research** is a systematic, objective process used to pose questions about variables and the relationships among variables and then to measure and test those relationships using precise statistical methods. This is accomplished by following a five-phase process that guides the research. *(Objective 1)*

- In Phase 1, conceptualization of the research problem, the researcher formulates a problem, reviews the literature, develops a theoretical framework, and formulates the variables. *(Objective 2)*

  - **Research problems** arise from gaps in the state of the science. A **problem statement** describes the problem, its significance, and the need to study the problem. The **purpose** states the study intent.

  - A **literature review** and **theoretical framework** form a foundation for the study. The review of the literature provides a comprehensive overview of any materials relevant to the topic under study.

  - The theoretical framework forms a frame of reference for the study using a relevant **theory** that will explain the phenomena under study.

  - **Research questions** or **hypotheses** are used to identify the variables to be studied. In quantitative research, concepts are called **variables** and may be classified as **independent**, **dependent**, or **extraneous** in nature. **Conceptual** and **operational definitions** are then delineated for identified variables.

- In Phase 2, design the study, the researcher selects a study design, identifies the population and sample, and chooses instruments for data collection. *(Objective 3)*
  - **Research designs** can be classified as experimental or non-experimental.
  - A **population** contains the participants of interest to a researcher and a **sample** is a representative piece of a population. **Generalizability** means that the study results from the sample can be applied to the population. **Probability samples** mathematically ensure a representative sample. There are four types of probability samples: simple random, stratified random, cluster, and systematic random. There are four types of **non-probability samples**: convenience, quota, purposive, and systematic.
  - **Instruments** collect **data**, measurable information about physiological, behavioral, or psychological phenomena. A good instrument must have **reliability** and **validity**. There are three types of reliability: internal consistency, stability, and equivalence, and three types of validity: content, criterion, and construct.
- In Phase 3, implement the design, the researcher addresses any ethical concerns, recruits participants, and collects the data. *(Objective 4)*
  - Study participants have rights and must be informed of the risks and benefits of the study. Institutional review boards (IRBs) are charged with the responsibility of ensuring that a research participant's rights are protected.
  - An informed consent indicates that an individual has been briefed on the study and has agreed to participate and is thus available to participate in the study.
  - The design is put into action as data is generated, collected, and recorded.
- In Phase 4, analyze and interpret the data, the researcher describes the sample and presents and interprets the findings. *(Objective 5)*
  - Researchers use **descriptive statistics** to describe the sample and answer the research question(s), and prove or disprove the hypotheses.
  - The three common ways to statistically describe data are frequencies, measures of central tendency, and measures of dispersion.
  - Statistics are run to answer the research questions/hypotheses and this produces the study **findings**, which are interpreted and placed in context of the literature.
- In Phase 5, use the results, the researcher suggests **implications** of the results and **disseminates** the findings so that research consumers can use them in the practice of nursing. This in turn generates new problems in need of research, which starts the process anew. *(Objective 6)*

Now that you understand the quantitative research process, it is time for you to see whether you can apply what you have learned.

STUDENT ACTIVITIES

1. Go to a recent issue of a research journal such as *Applied Nursing Research* or *Clinical Nursing Research*. Select a quantitative research study (Hint: look for statistics in the analysis section). Now read the article and see if you can locate evidence of the key steps in Phase 1.

    a. What problem is being investigated? Is there a problem statement and/or a purpose listed?

    b. Look at the literature review (Hint: it is often labeled background or introduction). Did this help you better understand the context of the study? Did they use a theoretical framework?

    c. What variables are being tested (Hint: look for a research question or hypotheses)? Can you locate the definitions of terms?

2. Keep reading your article as you look for evidence associated with the steps in Phase 2 of a research study.

    a. Locate the research design. Can you determine whether it is an experimental or non-experimental study?

    b. Locate the sample. What sampling technique was used? Is that a probability or non-probability technique? How many participants were in the sample?

    c. What instruments were used to measure the variables? Can you tell if the instruments are reliable? Valid?

3. Keep reading your article as you look for evidence associated with the steps in Phase 3 of a research study.

    a. Were the rights of the participants protected? Is there any evidence that IRB approval was obtained? Was an informed consent used?

    b. Does the study describe the data collection procedure?

4. Keep reading your article as you look for evidence associated with the steps in Phases 4 and 5 of a research study.

    a. Can you locate a sample description? What statistics were used to describe the sample?

    b. Find the answers to the research problem that was posed. Are the results clearly stated in narrative format?

    c. Did the researchers discuss how their findings related back to the literature?

    d. Did the researcher discuss how the study findings could be used in nursing practice? Were recommendations for further research made?

Pearson Nursing Student Resources

Find additional review materials at

www.nursing.pearsonhighered.com

Prepare for success with additional NCLEX®-style practice questions, interactive assignments and activities, web links, animations and videos, and more!

REFERENCES

Bennett, J.A., H.M. Young, L.M. Nail, K. Winters-Stone, and G. Hanson. 2008. A telephone-only motivational intervention to increase physical activity in rural adults. *Nursing Research, 57*(1): 24–32.

Cheung, R., V.Y. Cureton, and D.L. Canaham. 2006. Quality of life in adolescents with type 1 diabetes who participate in diabetes camp. *The Journal of School Nursing, 22*(1): 53–58.

Chlan, L.L., W.C. Engeland, A. Anthony, and J. Guttormson. 2007. Influence of music on the stress response in patients receiving mechanical ventilatory support: A pilot study. *American Journal of Critical Care, 16*(2): 141–145.

Cohen, L.S, L. Sedhorn, M. Salifu, and E. Friedman. 2007. Inpatient diabetes management: Examining morning practice in an acute care setting. *The Diabetes Educator, 33*(3): 483–492.

Gilje, F.L., P.M. Klose, and C.J. Birger. 2007. Critical clinical competencies in undergraduate psychiatric-mental health nursing. *Journal of Nursing Educaion, 46*(11): 522–526.

Hertig, V.L., K.C. Cain, M.E. Jarrett, R.L. Burr, and M.M. Heitkemper. 2007. Daily distress and gastrointestinal symptoms in women with irritable bowel syndrome. *Nursing Research, 56*(6): 399–406.

International Association for the Study of Pain. 1994. Task force on taxonomy classification of chronic pain. In H. Mersky & N. Bogduk (eds.), *Classification of chronic pain: description of chronic pain syndromes and definition of pain terms* (2nd ed.) (pp. 209–214). Seattle, WA: IASP Press.

Langford, R. 2001. *Navigating the maze of nursing research.* St. Louis, MO: Mosby.

Lazenbatt, A. and R. Freeman. 2006. Recognizing and reporting child physical abuse: a survey of primary healthcare professionals. *Journal of Advanced Nursing, 56*(3): 227–236.

Leonhardt, C., S. Keller, J. Chenot, J. Luckmann, H. Basler, K. Wegscheider, et al. 2008. TTM-based motivational counselling does not increase physical activity of low back pain patients in a primary care setting—A cluster-randomized controlled trial. Patient Education and Counseling, 70(1): 50–60.

Manojlovich, M. 2005. Predictors of professional nursing practice behaviors in hospital settings. *Nursing Research, 54*(1): 41–47.

McFarlane, J.M., J.Y. Groff, J.A. O'Brien, and K. Watson. 2006. Secondary prevention of intimate partner violence: a randomized controlled trial. *Nursing Research, 55*(1): 1–10.

Rabin, C. and N. Tabak. 2006. Healthy participants in phase 1 clinical trials: the quality of their decision to take part. *Journal of Clinical Nursing, 15*(8): 971–979.

Quantitative Research Approaches

CHAPTER OUTLINE

CHAPTER OBJECTIVES

1. Discuss the expanded definition of quantitative research.
2. Describe four major means of classifying quantitative research.
3. Identify the key feature that separates experimental and non-experimental designs.
4. Discuss distinguishing characteristics between true experimental, quasi-experimental, and pre-experimental design types.
5. Describe the strengths and weaknesses of experimental research.
6. Discuss the reasons for using non-experimental designs in a research study.

KEY TERMS

Applied research (p. 111)

Basic research (p. 126)

Control group (p. 116)

Cross-sectional study (p. 113)

Descriptive study (p. 112)

Experimental research (p. 114)

Explanatory study (p. 126)

Exploratory study (p. 112)

Intervention study (p. 115)

Longitudinal study (p. 113)

Manipulation (p. 114)

Non-experimental research (p. 115)

Predictive study (p. 112)

Pre-experimental design (p. 120)

Prospective study (p. 114)

Quasi-experimental design (p. 118)

Random assignment (p. 116)

Randomized control trial (RCT) (p. 114)

Retrospective study (p. 114)

True experimental design (p. 115)

ABSTRACT

Quantitative research is a structured phase-by-phase, step-by-step process used to describe, explore, explain, and predict measurable conditions. Quantitative research can be classified in numerous ways, including reasons conducted, purpose, time factors, and research design. The experimental or non-experimental design classification is a particularly useful categorization that allows us to determine whether the study is testing a specific nursing intervention that may produce useful evidence to change or alter nursing practice.

This chapter is designed to give you a more detailed examination of a number of ways by which we typically classify and describe quantitative research studies. We will then examine experimental and non-experimental research in greater detail by describing sub-classifications of the two and providing specific examples from the research literature.

Quantitative Research Revisited

We introduced you to the concept of research in Chapter 3 and expanded the concept in Chapter 4 as we differentiated the two major traditions of qualitative and quantitative research. Chapter 5 focused on quantitative research and the quantitative research process. Let's now expand our definition again by exploring specific ways of classifying quantitative research.

Quantitative research is a very structured phase-by-phase, step-by-step process used to describe, explore, explain, and predict measurable conditions. It begins with the conceptualization of a researchable problem which is grounded in a theoretical base derived from relevant literature. Researchers form research questions or hypotheses to guide their inquiry. They then design the study and select the sample and instruments. They collect data, analyze and interpret it, and disseminate the findings so they can be used in practice. This process provides us with clear answers to precise questions for a specified sample of participants. It also plants the seeds for future research problems that need attention.

Quantitative Research Classifications

There are a number of ways to describe quantitative research. We are going to explore the most common classifications.

Quantitative research may be classified in one of four ways: the motivation for conducting the research, the purpose or aim of the research, the point and time span of data collection, and the research design. Box 6-1 shows these classifications.

Consider This ...

Before reading about each classification system, look at Box 6-1 and determine what you think the classifications might mean. Then read the sections below and see how close you came.

Reasons Conducted

Research can be classified according to the motivation propelling the conduct of the research. **Basic research**, also known as pure or fundamental research, is a search for "knowledge for knowledge's sake." It is conducted to establish or extend the knowledge

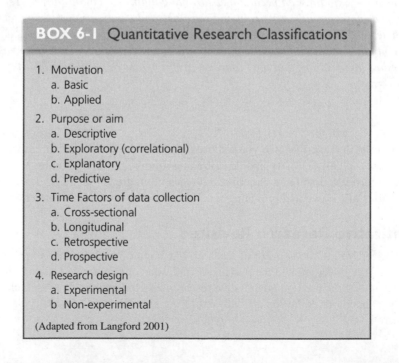

BOX 6-1 Quantitative Research Classifications

1. Motivation
   a. Basic
   b. Applied

2. Purpose or aim
   a. Descriptive
   b. Exploratory (correlational)
   c. Explanatory
   d. Predictive

3. Time Factors of data collection
   a. Cross-sectional
   b. Longitudinal
   c. Retrospective
   d. Prospective

4. Research design
   a. Experimental
   b Non-experimental

(Adapted from Langford 2001)

> ## BOX 6-2 Example of Basic Nursing Research
>
> Hastings-Tolsma (2006) conducted basic research to propose and test a theory of diversity of human field pattern. The purpose of the study was "(a) to determine the validity of Rogers' proposition that individuals have the capacity to participate in the process of change, and (b) to validate the construct of diversity of human field pattern" (p. 34).
>
> This study is clearly aimed at testing and extending a construct described in Martha Rogers' nursing theory of the Science of Unitary Human Beings. While the findings have ultimate implications for the theoretical understanding of nursing practice, this research study makes no attempt to solve a particular problem in current clinical practice.

base in a discipline. For nursing, that might include the exploration of fundamental concepts and theories that form the foundation or base for the discipline of nursing. Basic research is not aimed at solving problems in nursing practice and the findings from such research studies seldom have immediate practical applications. They do, however, provide new ways to view key concepts or theories that are fundamental in nursing. See an example of basic research in Box 6-2.

Basic research is not conducted often in nursing, and funding for basic research is often difficult to obtain. Many nurse scientists would argue that basic research forms the foundation for applied research and provides the underlying understanding needed for real progress and growth in the profession. George Smoot, an astrophysicist and Nobel prize-winner for physics, said in part, "If we only did applied research, we would still be making better spears" (Lawrence Berkeley National Laboratory 2007).

The overall goal of applied research is to improve the human condition. **Applied research** is done to discover answers to practical problems in our everyday personal or professional worlds. It might include evaluating or testing a specified intervention, procedure, product, or program. Because nursing is a practice-based discipline, the majority of the research in various nursing research journals is applied research. As a consumer of nursing research who desires to improve clinical practice, you will be most interested in applied research. Box 6-3 shows just one example of applied research. There is an entire nursing research journal devoted to this branch of research which is appropriately entitled *Applied Nursing Research*.

> ## BOX 6-3 Example of Applied Research
>
> Yoo, Kim, Hur, and Kim (2011) conducted applied research to determine whether an animation distraction technique would work to reduce pain response in preschool children undergoing venipuncture. They found that the distraction intervention reduced self-report, behavioral, and physiological pain responses in the treatment group.
>
> This study provides answers that can easily be used by nurses in daily practice.

Purpose or Aim

Quantitative studies are often classified by purpose or aim. In the beginning of this chapter, we stated that quantitative research was used to describe, explore, explain, and predict. This method of classification identifies the general purpose of a research study. As you will see,

BOX 6-4 Examples of Descriptive Studies

Example 1: A study by Miller, Guo, and Rodseth (2011) was designed to look at bladder habits of healthy women in the community. This study described data clusters about intake, output, and voiding habits collected in a 3-day self-report voiding diary. This study was done in preparation for further research which would tailor and then test interventions to decrease the risk for incontinence.

Example 2: A study by Cohen et al. (2007) was conducted to describe the current practices of managing morning diabetes in hospitalized acute care and to identify the effects of that management. This study was done to determine whether current hospital practices for diabetes management needed modification.

the names in this category are very descriptive of the study purpose. A **descriptive study**, for example, describes identified concepts that are being studied. It focuses on such attributes as the incidence, prevalence, magnitude, or characteristics of the concepts. It might ask research questions such as *How often does the concept occur?* or *What are the characteristics identified with the concept?* Such studies are frequently conducted to obtain needed detail on a concept for further research study, as the examples in Box 6-4 show.

An **exploratory study** goes beyond the description of concepts to explore the relationships between the identified concept(s) and other concepts, as the examples in Box 6-5 show. They are also referred to as correlational studies. It might ask research questions such as *What concepts are related to the concept of interest?* or *Are there differences in categories of a concept?*

BOX 6-5 Examples of Exploratory Studies

Example 1: A study by Im et al. (2007) explored the differences in males and females and in four ethnic groups on cancer pain experiences. The research questions of interest were whether differences existed for men versus women and among Caucasians, Hispanics, African Americans, and/or Asian Americans on perceptions of cancer pain. So this study is exploring group differences on the concept of interest "pain".

Example 2: A study by Cuellar, Hanlon, and Ratcliff (2011) explored the relationship between serum iron levels in the body and RLS symptom severity, sleep quality, daytime sleepiness, depression, fatigue, and quality of life for participants. This study is exploring relationships among iron stores and several other concepts.

Explanatory studies explain. These studies attempt to understand why certain concept(s) occur and explain why concepts are related. They may search for a specific cause-and-effect relationship between concepts or sort out and diagram the way that multiple concepts interrelate. Such studies may also try to explain how concepts are linked to a particular theory. Box 6-6 includes some examples of explanatory studies. Research questions may ask *Does one factor cause another factor?* or *Does this theory explain the behavior of a specific concept(s)?*

BOX 6-6 Examples of Explanatory Studies

Example 1: A study by Weinert, Cudney, Comstock, and Bansal (2011) used control and treatment groups of participants to examine whether a computer-based intervention could increase psychosocial adaptation of middle aged rural women with chronic health conditions. This study is looking at a cause-and-effect connection between the computer-based treatment and psychologic adaptation.

Example 2: A study by Olbrys (2011) studied the effects of patient education for women scheduled for colposcopy and their compliance to treatment recommendations. This study examined whether education affected compliance to treatment. It was trying to examine whether education was an effective means in getting patients to be compliant.

A **predictive study** is designed to determine whether researchers can use the occurrence of a concept or concepts to predict changes in another concept, as you can see from the examples in Box 6-7. Research questions may ask *If concept X occurs will concept Y occur?* or *If concept X changes will concept Y change in an expected manner?* If we can predict certain concepts or factors, we may be able to exert some control over those factors.

BOX 6-7 Examples of Predictive Studies

Example 1: A study by Ham (2011) attempted to predict health related quality of life in low income middle aged women using sociodemographic, biomedical, psychosocial, and medical-care factors. They were looking at factors which would predict quality of life so that they might be modified.

Example 2: A study by McCullagh, Ronis, and Lusk (2010) developed a model to predict the use of effective hearing protection and then tested the model to determine whether it would predict the use of hearing protection in a group of farmers. Findings supporting such a model would be useful in designing interventions to increase farmers' hearing protector use.

Time Factors of Data Collection

Research is sometimes described by the point at which the data were collected. When data is collected at a single point in time it is considered a **cross-sectional study**. That means that the concepts in the study are measured once and the data are collected during that time period. This type of study thus examines the status of concepts at a fixed point in time. A **longitudinal study** collects data from a number of points in time. This data collection can take place over months or years. Such studies are frequently used to describe how concepts change over time or to examine the sequence in which concepts or events occur. For example, researchers might be interested in studying whether the length of time that a patient has been diagnosed with hypertension affects medication adherence. In a cross-sectional study, the researcher might locate a group of patients in a hypertension clinic, and use one afternoon to collect data on how long they have had hypertension and on how well they take their medication. In a longitudinal study a researcher might locate a group of newly diagnosed patients and follow them over a period of years while periodically checking their medication adherence.

There is a longstanding longitudinal research study that is focused on women's health which uses nurses as participants. It is known as the Nurse's Health Study (NHS) and is conducted by researchers at Harvard University. The original study was begun in 1976 and expanded in 1989. They have collected comprehensive health data about cancer, heart disease, diabetes, and a variety of lifestyle factors on over 238,000 nurse participants over a 22 to 35 year period of time. Another study expansion (NHS3) was started in 2012. Check out their web site at www.channing.harvard.edu/nhs/. If you would like to be a participant in Nurses' Health Study 3 (NHS3) go to the study site at www.nhs3.org.

Research can also be described by looking at the point in time at which the data was generated. A **prospective study** collects data on factors or events as they unfold. It often starts with a presumed cause and moves forward in time to a presumed effect. A **retrospective study** collects data on factors or events that occurred before the research study began. It may start with a present factor and then examine that factor in light of pre-existing factors. For example, researchers might be interested in whether the ingestion of caffeine during pregnancy influences miscarriage rates. In a prospective study, the researchers would measure caffeine intake in a group of women over the course of their pregnancies and then record the number of miscarriages that occurred. In a retrospective study, the researcher might start with a group of women who had suffered a miscarriage and ask them about their caffeine intake during their pregnancy.

Consider This . . .

Do you think quantitative studies can be classified in more than one category simultaneously? Why or why not?

Research Design

Perhaps the most common and most useful way to describe and classify quantitative research is by the research design that was used. There are two major research design categories: experimental and non-experimental. In **experimental research**, the researcher administers an intervention or treatment to a group of participants to see whether that treatment causes changes to the concept under study. This is known as a **manipulation**. The researcher manipulates one factor under study to see how that manipulation will change or affect another factor under study. In medical research, and increasingly in nursing research, experimental designs are referred to as a controlled trial or a **randomized controlled trial (RCT)**. In truth an RCT is a type of experimental research that follows a true experimental design and uses a large sample collected from multiple sites and settings. Box 6-8 gives examples of two experimental studies.

BOX 6-8 Examples of Experimental Studies

Example 1: A study by Bennett et al. (2008) examined "whether a telephone-only motivation interviewing intervention would increase daily physical activity of rural adults" (p. 24). The researchers are using a treatment (telephone interview) to see if it will impact the amount of physical activity.

Example 2: Another study by Nyamathi et al. (2007) examined whether a nurse case management intervention would improve adherence to a tuberculosis medication regimen in homeless adults. Again you see that the researchers are using a treatment (case management) to see whether it will impact medication adherence.

BOX 6-9 Examples of Non-Experimental Studies

Example 1: A study by Im et al. (2007) explored the differences in males and females and in four ethnic groups on their cancer pain experiences. Researchers are looking at cancer pain experiences and seeing whether these experiences are affected by gender or ethnicity. Note that the researchers are not manipulating gender or ethnicity because they cannot be manipulated. Instead the researchers are studying the factors as they occur.

Example 2: A study by Miller, Guo, and Rodseth (2011) was designed to look at bladder habits of healthy women in the community. This study described data clusters about intake, output, and voiding habits collected in a 3-day self-report voiding diary. This study was done in preparation for further research which would tailor and then test interventions to decrease the risk for incontinence.

In **non-experimental research**, the researchers act as observers but do not administer a treatment. There is no manipulation. The concepts are observed or studied as they occur naturally. For example, in the Bennett study in Box 6-8, suppose the researchers were simply evaluating the care that was routinely administered by home health nurses in relation to the amount of physical activity in rural adults. The study would then be classified as non-experimental because the researchers were not introducing any new intervention. Box 6-9 has additional examples of non-experimental studies.

As you may have suspected, studies may be described by more than one of these classifications. So you might see a study described as cross-sectional and non-experimental, explanatory and experimental, or descriptive and longitudinal, to give just a few examples. (See Example 1 in Box 6-4 and Example 2 in Box 6-9.)

Experimental and Non-Experimental Designs

Now that you have a general idea about experimental and non-experimental designs and have viewed examples of each design category, let's examine each in more depth.

Experimental Designs

Researchers use experimental designs to examine cause-and-effect relationships between variables and these are often known as **intervention studies**. An experimental design can be very useful in providing information about specific nursing interventions and protocols. They may be further classified as true experimental, quasi-experimental, or pre-experimental in nature. These sub-classifications contain a number of specific designs (Campbell and Stanley 1963), and are illustrated in Figure 6-1. The listed designs are the ones that you are most likely to see when reading the research literature.

TRUE EXPERIMENTAL DESIGNS. **True experimental designs** are the strongest form of experimental design and are characterized by three key features: 1) manipulation, 2) control, and 3) random assignment. Researchers use these three properties to try to ensure that the independent variable is the factor that causes the change in the dependent variable. You know from previous discussion that manipulation involves an intervention or treatment that the researcher administers. This treatment is given to attempt to produce a change in the dependent variable.

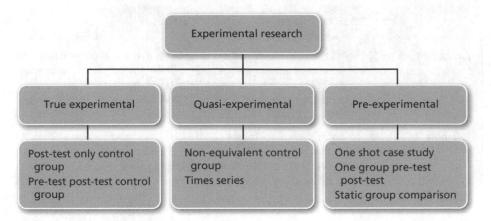

■ FIGURE 6-1 Experimental Design Classifications

To make sure it is the intervention that causes the change, rather than some extraneous factor, the researcher also applies controls to the experiment. This usually entails placing some of the participants in a **control group** that does not receive the study intervention. However, control group members often receive a placebo treatment or some alternative treatment such as the usual method of care. For example, suppose a researcher wants to test the effects of a new gel mattress overlay on prevention of pressure ulcers in nursing home patients. The intervention group would be placed on the gel mattress and the control group would use the alternating-pressure air mattress that is standard on that particular care unit. After administering the intervention, the researcher can then measure the dependent variable in all participants in the sample and compare the group that received no intervention (control group) to the group that received the intervention (treatment group). If the dependent variable differs between the two groups, then the researcher can infer that the intervention caused the difference. In our example, the researcher measures pressure conditions for the sample of nursing home residents that are on the special gel mattresses (intervention) versus the residents who are on the air mattresses (control). If the intervention group displays less evidence of pressure ulcers (dependent variable) than the control group, then the gel mattress would be seen as the more effective mattress in reducing pressure and thus preventing pressure ulcers.

When dividing the sample into control and treatment groups, the researcher wants each group's participants to be as similar as possible. This will minimize the chances that an extraneous characteristic such as age, gender, or ethnicity will affect the results. For example, in our mattress overlay study, if one group included mainly obese people and the other group had mostly underweight or normal weight people, the weight differences might influence the amount of pressure exerted by the mattress overlays, calling the research results into question. This brings us to the concept of **random assignment**, the final key feature of a true experimental design. Random assignment is used to equalize the two groups and to prevent extraneous factors from exerting an influence on the dependent variable. When the process of random assignment is used, every participant in the sample has an equal chance of being placed in either the treatment or the control group. Random assignment is also used to ensure that each group has an equal chance of being designated as the treatment group. (Note: Do not confuse the term *random assignment* with the term *random selection*. Random assignment refers to the placement of sample participants into a group. Random selection or random sampling is a probability sampling method used to select a sample from a population and was discussed in Chapter 5.)

Consider This . . .

What is the one design characteristic that is always present in an experimental study and distinguishes experimental from non-experimental studies?

When a research study employs a true experimental design, it offers maximum protection against bias and ensures that any changes in the dependent variable are indeed caused by the independent variable. Box 6-10 provides examples of two studies that illustrate the three key features of true experimental research.

In Example 1, the phrase *motivational intervention (MI)* alerts the reader to the fact that this is an experimental study. MI is the manipulation. The article clearly states that control and intervention groups were used and that the participants were randomly assigned to these groups. A fuller description of the manipulation can be seen in the description of the intervention that was administered. Now examine Example 2. Can you spot evidence of the three key characteristics of a true experimental study?

BOX 6-10 Examples of Key Features in True Experimental Designs

Example 1: A Telephone-Only Motivational Intervention to Increase Physical Activity in Rural Adults (Bennett et al. 2008)

". . . participants were randomized to intervention or control group using a computer-generated randomization list . . . Participants in the [motivational] intervention (MI) group received a telephone call from the study physical activity counselor . . . This telephone call was intended as a planning and goal-setting session . . . The call included guidelines for safety, such as warming up and cooling down, and a discussion of perceived exertion in terms of maintaining moderate levels of exercise . . . Control group participants were telephoned monthly and asked about their physical activity using a prescribed set of five questions in a script with no MI content" (pp. 25–26).

Example 2: Efficacy of Nurse Case-Managed Intervention for Latent Tuberculosis among Homeless Subsamples (Nyamathi et al. 2007)

"Homeless adults were advised of the study by . . . flyers posted in the 12 sites. These sites were randomized into the intervention and control [groups] . . . Interested persons visited the research nurses, . . . located at the neighborhood clinic a few blocks from their shelters . . . In both the intervention and control programs, homeless adults were required to present to the clinic twice a week over a period of 6 months . . . Participants in the intervention program attended eight comprehensive educational and skills training modules over the 6-month study period in small groups of four to five at a time . . . Information was provided on TB and HIV infection and risk reduction; strategies to improve self-esteem, coping, self management, and communication skills; and training in problem solving to implement behavior change and to develop relationships and social networks to maintain behavior change . . . For the control program, one 20-minute TB and HIV education session was delivered" (pp. 34–35).

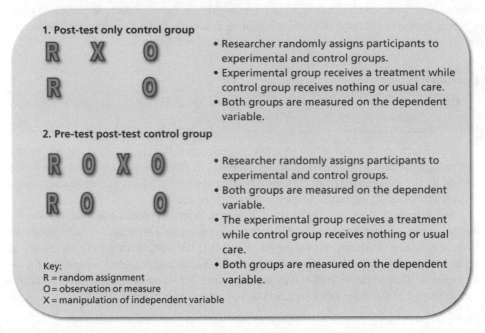

1. Post-test only control group

R   X   O
R   O

• Researcher randomly assigns participants to experimental and control groups.
• Experimental group receives a treatment while control group receives nothing or usual care.
• Both groups are measured on the dependent variable.

2. Pre-test post-test control group

R   O   X   O
R   O   O

• Researcher randomly assigns participants to experimental and control groups.
• Both groups are measured on the dependent variable.
• The experimental group receives a treatment while control group receives nothing or usual care.
• Both groups are measured on the dependent variable.

Key:
R = random assignment
O = observation or measure
X = manipulation of independent variable

■ **FIGURE 6-2** Types of True Experimental Designs

There are two common true experimental designs: 1) post-test only control group and 2) pre-test post-test control group, as shown in Figure 6-2. Both use a control group and an intervention group and both use random assignment of participants to the groups. The only difference lies in when the dependent variable is measured. In the *post-test only control group design*, the dependent variable is measured for both groups after the intervention is administered. In the *pre-test post-test control group design*, the dependent variable is measured for both groups both before and after the intervention is administered. The first, or pre-test, measure is often referred to as a baseline measure. When you peruse the research literature and are reading a study that employs a true experimental design, it is likely to be one of these two designs.

QUASI-EXPERIMENTAL DESIGNS. All experimental designs use manipulation. However, some cannot use control groups or random assignment to groups because it may not be feasible for the sample of participants selected for the study. For example, if participants in one group might influence outcomes of the participants in the second group, researchers might have the control group on one hospital unit and the experimental group on another to prevent cross contamination between the two groups. When a research design does not include control groups or uses control groups with no random assignment, it is called a **quasi-experimental design**. A quasi-experimental design must then use other means of control to ensure that the study results are valid and non-biased. The strength of these studies is determined by the alternative control measures that the researcher used to correct for the lack of a control group or random assignment.

When only one group is used, the researcher often strengthens the design by taking several measures of the dependent variable both before and after the intervention.

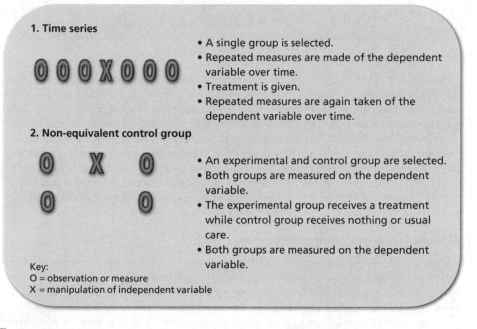

1. Time series

O O O X O O O

- A single group is selected.
- Repeated measures are made of the dependent variable over time.
- Treatment is given.
- Repeated measures are again taken of the dependent variable over time.

2. Non-equivalent control group

O   X   O

O   O

- An experimental and control group are selected.
- Both groups are measured on the dependent variable.
- The experimental group receives a treatment while control group receives nothing or usual care.
- Both groups are measured on the dependent variable.

Key:
O = observation or measure
X = manipulation of independent variable

■ **FIGURE 6-3** Types of Quasi-Experimental Designs

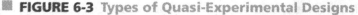

This is known as a *time series design*. Figure 6-3 shows a diagram of this design, while Example 1 in Box 6-11 gives an example of the time series design used in a study. Note the researchers' clear description of the design and the rationale they give for not using a two-group design.

When random assignment is not possible, researchers employ a *non-equivalent control group design*. This is a two-group design with a control and an intervention group that uses pre-test and post-test measures of the dependent variable. However, the groups were not randomly assigned (see Figure 6-3). You will note that it looks just like the second true experimental design in Figure 6-2 but without random assignment to groups.

A smart researcher will try to make sure that the two groups are similar on key characteristics such as age, gender, or disease process. When reading research, check for similarities by examining the descriptive statistics for key characteristics of the two groups. Researchers choosing this design may also employ statistical measures to check the two groups on the baseline measure of the dependent variable. If the two groups were at the same level on the dependent variable prior to the intervention, the reader can have more confidence in the comparison of differences in the two groups after the intervention. If the groups were different prior to the intervention, the researcher should use a statistical procedure as a correction factor. The reader should look for a description of how the pre-test results influenced statistical analysis to ensure that the study took appropriate action.

Example 2 in Box 6-11 shows a non-equivalent control group quasi-experimental design used in an actual research study. Note the description of the design and the rationale for the design. It is also important to note that the researchers used statistical measures to determine whether the groups were similar on baseline measures.

BOX 6-11 Examples of Quasi-Experimental Designs

Example 1: Time series design

"The purpose of this study was to test the effectiveness and feasibility of using an audio-visual, simplified Tai Chi exercise module to enhance and maintain the health of long-term care facility residents. A quasi-experimental, one-group, time-series design was used. Data were collected six times (twice before the intervention; four times after intervention started) at three-month interval . . . The intervention was conducted in two stages: (1) instructor-led STEP for the first six months and (2) video-guided STEP for the next six months. Performing the intervention in two stages within one group rather than with two groups using two different intervention methods was necessary because Tai Chi instruction delivered in audiovisual format (a video tape) can only be implemented once a participant is already familiar with Tai Chi movements" (Chen et al. 2007, pp. 156–157).

Example 2: Non-equivalent control group

"A quasi-experimental prospective study of patients with hip fracture was performed in which standard care was given to a comparison group and compared with an ICP-led intervention was given to a study group . . . A sample of 56 patients with hip fracture admitted to hospital from October 2003 to April 2004 was used to collect data for the comparison group. After a 7-month period that was used to develop and implement the ICP, data were collected from 56 patients with hip fracture who were cared for within an ICP framework" (Olsson et al. 2007, p. 117). [The two groups were statistically compared and were equivalent.]

"The randomized controlled trial design is considered the 'gold standard' in evaluating interventions; yet, its use can be limited by ethical and practical concerns. One of these concerns is the difficulty for nursing staff to work within two care systems at the same time. The present study was . . . quasi-experimental . . . A disadvantage of this design is that it precludes conclusions being the true effects of an intervention, i.e. knowing whether the between-group differences are due to the intervention or to other unknown factors . . . To the best of our knowledge, no changes took place in the hospital during the study period. Further, no routines or procedures were changed . . ." (Olsson et al. 2007, p. 122).

PRE-EXPERIMENTAL DESIGNS. A study that employs manipulation but fails to use other control measures is known as a **pre-experimental design**. This design is very weak and is open to many sources of bias. As noted in Figure 6-4, there are three pre-experimental designs. The first is known as a *one shot case study*. In this study the researcher administers an intervention to a group of participants and then measures the dependent variable. In this design there is no way to know what change, if any, occurred and whether the change was caused by the intervention or by other factors. The second design is a *one group pre-test post-test*, which attempts to examine a change in the dependent variable by taking a baseline measure of the dependent variable before the intervention. However, changes cannot be attributed to the intervention in this design as the changes could have occurred as a result of other factors in the environment.

The third design is a *static group comparison*. In this design the researchers use two groups but do not take baseline measures of the dependent variable so there is no way to know whether the groups started out at the same level on the dependent variable.

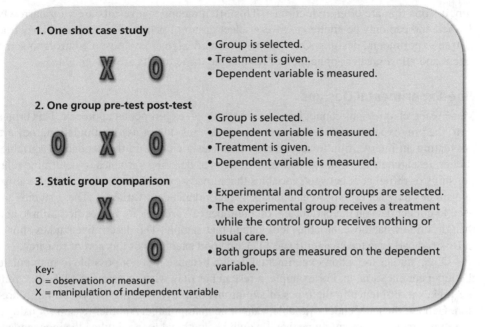

1. **One shot case study**

X   O

- Group is selected.
- Treatment is given.
- Dependent variable is measured.

2. **One group pre-test post-test**

O   X   O

- Group is selected.
- Dependent variable is measured.
- Treatment is given.
- Dependent variable is measured.

3. **Static group comparison**

X   O

O

- Experimental and control groups are selected.
- The experimental group receives a treatment while the control group receives nothing or usual care.
- Both groups are measured on the dependent variable.

Key:
O = observation or measure
X = manipulation of independent variable

■ **FIGURE 6-4** Types of Pre-Experimental Designs

Note that this design looks just like the first true experimental design that is illustrated in Figure 6-2 but without random assignment to groups.

Results from pre-experimental designs must be interpreted and used with extreme caution. They may, however, provide evidence that further study is needed in a given area. You will seldom see these designs reported in the published literature. If you do see one of these designs, remember that the reported findings are suspect. So, unless there is supportive evidence from other more strongly designed quasi- or true experimental studies, pre-experimental studies should not be used as evidence to change practice.

STRENGTHS AND WEAKNESSES OF EXPERIMENTAL DESIGNS. Experimental research is often viewed as the pinnacle of scientific research. True experimental designs, often referred to as randomized controlled trials or RCTs, are the most powerful method available for testing cause-and-effect relationships. They tell us whether specified interventions such as gel mattresses, case management, or motivational interviewing produce a change in identified dependent variables such as pressure ulcers, physical activity, or adherence to a TB medication regimen. True experimental designs yield the highest quality of evidence for nursing practice, allowing us to change our nursing practice with confidence. Nurses can institute interventions that have been tested under the most highly controlled conditions and found to produce a change. Evidence that is produced from multiple studies or from studies at multiple sites can be used even more confidently.

Experimental research does have its limitations, however. It does not allow for the examination of complex issues with multiple factors in play. The very requirements for a good experimental study create limits. The process itself requires that a very small number of variables be studied under very tightly controlled conditions. These conditions seldom reflect true life and variables seldom occur only in the manner tested. This leads to conclusions that are often reductionist. This often means that results are very narrowly defined and can only be applied to a very select group of people. This is particularly true of true experimental designs. Quasi-experimental designs may loosen controls to some extent and allow greater application of results, but those results are less conclusive.

Non-Experimental Designs

Many research questions cannot be addressed using an experimental approach. This brings us to the non-experimental design. Since these designs do not use manipulation, they are not testing an intervention to see whether it causes a change in the dependent variable. Rather, researchers use non-experimental designs to describe variables or determine relationships or differences between variables that already exist in the environment. Descriptive studies may not even designate independent or dependent variables. These studies are used to collect data on the parameters of a number of variables for a specified sample and then describe what those variables look like in that sample. The descriptive studies shown in Box 6-4 earlier in the chapter (page 112) are good examples of this sort of research.

Other studies use a non-experimental design because it is not possible to manipulate the independent variable. For example, a researcher may wish to determine whether gender makes a difference in the types of symptoms displayed during a myocardial infarction. Gender, the independent variable, cannot be manipulated. Another reason for using a non-experimental study might be that it would be unethical to manipulate the independent variable. For example, suppose a researcher wanted to examine the effects that hormone supplements have on morbidity and mortality for women experiencing menopause. The independent variable here is the use or non-use of hormone supplements and it would be unethical to force women to take the hormones or to withhold hormones from women who desired them. A non-experimental study would allow the researcher to compare a hormone group to a non-hormone group. The researchers did not manipulate the independent variable of hormone choice; the participants made the choice before their involvement in the study.

A third reason for not manipulating the independent variable is because the intervention has already occurred. If researchers suspect a cause-and-effect relationship, they might first explore the variables using a non-experimental design to provide evidence that the more expensive experimental design is justified. For example, a nurse practitioner might notice that some physicians in a particular hospital prescribe one type of dressing for treatment of pressure ulcers while other physicians prescribe another type. Based on her observations while caring for these patients, she suspects that the second, more expensive type of dressing is more effective. However, before recommending an experimental study to determine the effectiveness of the two dressing types, she first works with the research nurse to compare past patients who had already been treated with one of the two dressing types. Together, they pull charts on patients who have been treated for stage one or stage two pressure ulcers, and split the charts into two groups based on dressing type. They then check the success of the treatment by checking the amount of time required for healing. To tighten controls on the two groups, they compare factors such as age, gender, ethnicity, and general debility. They compare the two groups and find that the second dressing type indeed shows a quicker healing time. This provides sufficient evidence to recommend the conduct of an experimental study.

A fourth reason to use a non-experimental design is when the researcher wishes to examine the relationships between multiple variables to determine whether there is a set of independent variables that can predict a change in a particular dependent variable or set of dependent variables. The researcher here is less concerned with cause and effect and more concerned with the complex interactions among multiple variables. Many of these studies use sophisticated and complex statistical analyses such as path analysis or multiple regression to predict or test theories of causality.

Consider This ...

Do you think an experimental design is better than a non-experimental design? Why or why not?

Box 6-12 shows some examples of non-experimental studies. Note particularly the language used to describe each non-experimental design; studies are seldom identified by the term *non-experimental*. Instead researchers might call them descriptive, retrospective, post hoc, correlational, or survey research. The reader may need to investigate to determine whether a study is non-experimental. The key factor is the lack of a treatment or intervention. When reading research, check to see whether a treatment or intervention was administered. If not, then the study is non-experimental.

BOX 6-12 Examples of Non-Experimental Designs

Example 1: Gender and Ethnic Differences in Cancer Pain Experience (Im et al. 2007)

This study used a cross-sectional survey design of 480 cancer patients in the United States to study gender and ethnic differences in the cancer pain experience. Data was collected via the internet using a questionnaire with multiple scales to assess pain perception.

Example 2: Inpatient diabetes management: Examining morning practice in an acute care setting (Cohen et al. 2007)

This study was described as "A descriptive, non-experimental research design" (p. 483) used to study the effect of the duration of time of blood glucose monitoring, insulin administration, and breakfast on the pre-lunch glucose levels.

Example 3: Pain-Sensitive Temperament and Post-Operative Pain (Kleiber et al. 2007)

This study described the relationship between pain sensitive temperament and self-report of pain intensity following surgery. Pain sensitive temperament was collected using a sensitivity temperament inventory on 60 adolescents with neuromuscular disorders who had had surgery at some time in the past 2.5 years. Pain intensity was collected from post op records in the medical record.

Example 4: The Effects of Acculturation on Asthma Burden in a Community Sample of Mexican American Schoolchildren (Martin et al. 2007)

This study "sought to determine whether low acculturation among Mexican American caregivers protects their children against asthma. Data were obtained from an observational study of urban pediatric asthma. Dependent variables were children's diagnosed asthma and total (diagnosed plus possible) asthma. Regression models were controlled for caregivers' level of acculturation, education, marital status, depression, life stress, and social support and children's insurance" (p. 1290).

In Example 1, the study is merely labeled as a cross-sectional survey design. However, the two independent variables can be identified as gender and ethnicity. So we know the study is non-experimental because these two variables cannot be manipulated. In Example 2, the design is clearly labeled as non-experimental. In Example 3, there was no direct description of the study design. However, the use of a retrospective approach is evident in the data collection description. A retrospective study cannot be experimental because it is impossible to impose a treatment on events that have already occurred. In Example 4, the study is simply described as observational. This tells us there was no intervention, only observation. Other clues that the study is non-experimental include the examination of the multiple independent variables, which for the most part cannot be manipulated, and the use of multiple regression statistics, which are used to examine relationships among multiple variables.

Non-experimental studies allow us to view multiple variables in action with one another. This can provide a better real world picture than a tightly controlled experimental design. The results, however, may not be as clear cut or directly interpretable as the results produced in experimental studies. Non-experimental studies can be used to provide evidence to support nursing practice. They allow us to view the behavior of non-manipulable variables as well as to examine the relationships among several variables simultaneously. They allow us to go back in time and examine variables that have already occurred. They can be useful in documenting the prevalence or nature of health-related conditions. However, they seldom provide sufficient evidence to promote a change in a specific nursing intervention on their own.

Take a look at the *Research in the News* feature on hearing loss in teenagers. What sort of research was conducted to reach the reported findings?

Research in the News

Study: 1 in 5 US Teenagers Has Slight Hearing Loss

BY CARLA K. JOHNSON,
AP Medical Writer © 2010 The Associated Press, Aug. 17, 2010, 8:34PM

CHICAGO—A stunning one in five teens has lost a little bit of hearing, and the problem has increased substantially in recent years, a new national study has found.

Some experts are urging teenagers to turn down the volume on their digital music players, suggesting loud music through earbuds may be to blame—although hard evidence is lacking. They warn that slight hearing loss can cause problems in school and set the stage for hearing aids in later life.

"Our hope is we can encourage people to be careful," said the study's senior author, Dr. Gary Curhan of Harvard-affiliated Brigham and Women's Hospital in Boston.

The researchers analyzed data on 12- to 19-year-olds from a nationwide health survey. They compared hearing loss in nearly 3,000 kids tested from 1988–94 to nearly 1,800 kids tested over 2005–06.

The prevalence of hearing loss increased from about 15 percent to 19.5 percent.

Most of the hearing loss was "slight," defined as inability to hear at 16 to 24 decibels—or sounds such as a whisper or rustling leaves. A teenager with slight hearing loss might not be able to hear water dripping or his mother whispering "good night."

Extrapolating to the nation's teens that would mean about 6.5 million with at least slight hearing loss.

Those with slight hearing loss "will hear all of the vowel sounds clearly, but might miss some of the consonant sounds" such as t, k and s, Curhan said.

"Although speech will be detectable, it might not be fully intelligible," he said.

While the researchers didn't single out iPods or any other device for blame, they found a significant increase in high-frequency hearing loss, which they said may indicate that noise caused the problems. And they cited a 2010 Australian study that linked use of personal listening devices with a 70 percent increased risk of hearing loss in children.

"I think the evidence is out there that prolonged exposure to loud noise is likely to be harmful to hearing, but that doesn't mean kids can't listen to MP3 players," Curhan said.

The study is based on data from the National Health and Nutrition Examination Survey conducted by a branch of the Centers for Disease Control and Prevention. The findings appear in Wednesday's Journal of the American Medical Association.

Here is a report on a research study that made headline news.

> Can you tell anything about how you would classify this study from this news report?

> Do we know if the researchers did an experimental study that would show that digital music players are causing the deafness? Or is this a non-experimental study that looks at relationships?

The answers are there—look at the key sentence:

They compared hearing loss in nearly 3,000 kids tested from 1988–94 to nearly 1,800 kids tested over 2005–06.

This tells us that researchers compared deafness levels in a sample of kids from one time period (they probably used a databank) with deafness levels in another sample of kids from a survey. So it is a non-experimental study and we don't know what caused the increase in hearing losses.

Check out the actual research study: Shargorodsky, J., S.G. Curhan, G.C. Curhan, and R. Eavey. 2010. Change in prevalence of hearing loss in us adolescents. *Journal of the American Medical Association*, 304(7): 772–778.

SUMMARY

In this chapter, you have examined a number of classifications for types of research and seen examples of each type from published research studies. Here is a summary of the key points in this chapter:

- Quantitative research is a highly structured research process used to answer questions about statistically measurable concepts. *(Objective 1)*

- Quantitative research can be classified in four ways: whether the research goal is **basic research** or **applied research**; whether the purpose is a **descriptive study, exploratory study, explanatory study,** or **predictive study**; whether the time factors involved in data collection are based on a **cross-sectional study,** a **longitudinal study**, or a **retrospective study**; and whether the research is **experimental research** or **non-experimental research.** *(Objective 2)*

- Experimental designs use **manipulation** as a means to examine cause-and-effect relationships while non-experimental designs do not use manipulation to study variables or their relationships. *(Objective 3)*

- Experimental designs are classified as true experimental, quasi-experimental, and pre-experimental. A **true experimental design** is characterized by manipulation, control, and **random assignment**. The two most common true experiments are post-test only control group designs and pre-test post-test control group designs. A **quasi-experimental design** uses manipulation but lacks either control or random assignment. Quasi-experiments may use a time series design or a non-equivalent control group. A **pre-experimental design** uses manipulation but lacks control and random assignment. A pre-experiment may be designed as a one shot case study, a one group pre-test post-test, or a static group comparison. *(Objective 4)*

- While experimental research offers researchers a powerful method for testing causal relationships, it falls short when it comes to examining complex, multi-factor issues. *(Objective 5)*

- **Non-experimental designs** do not manipulate variables. Researchers use non-experimental designs when they need to describe a variable or explore relationships or differences between variables that have already occurred. If researchers cannot manipulate the independent variable, then they use a non-experimental design. *(Objective 6)*

STUDENT ACTIVITIES

1. Look up some of the research studies cited as examples in the boxes in this chapter. Do not worry about being able to decipher them at this point. Can you tell why they are classified as they are?

2. Now choose some other quantitative research articles. Can you tell how to classify them as either experimental or non-experimental? What key terms might cue you in to the type of research design?

3. Now locate a true experimental article and a quasi-experimental article. What cues did you use to determine if they were a true experimental design versus a

quasi-experimental design? Do the studies you found match any of the true or quasi-experimental designs that we discussed in the chapter?

4. Which of the studies that you found might be useful to you in your clinical practice? How much faith would you place in the study results? Why?

Pearson Nursing Student Resources

Find additional review materials at

www.nursing.pearsonhighered.com

Prepare for success with additional NCLEX®-style practice questions, interactive assignments and activities, web links, animations and videos, and more!

REFERENCES

Bennett, J. A., H. M. Young, L. M. Nail, K. Winters-Stone, and G. Hanson. 2008. A telephone–only motivational intervention to increase physical activity in rural adults: a randomized controlled trial. *Nursing Research, 57*(1): 24–32.

Campbell, D. T. and J. Stanley. 1963. *Experimental and Quasi-experimental designs for research.* Chicago, IL: Rand McNally.

Chen, K., C. Li, J. Lin, W. Chen, H. Lin, and H. Wu. 2007. A feasible method to enhance and maintain the health of elderly living in long-term care facilities through long-term, simplified tai chi exercises. *Journal of Nursing Research, 15*(2): 156–163.

Cohen, L., L. Sedhom, M. Salifu, and E. Friedman. 2007. Examining morning practice in an acute care setting. *The Diabetes Educator, 3*(3): 483–493.

Cuellar, N., A. Hanlon, and S. Ratcliffe. 2011. The relationship with iron and health outcomes in persons with restless legs syndrome. *Clinical Nursing Research, 20*(2): 144–61.

Ham, O. 2011. Predictors of health-related quality of life among low-income midlife women. *Western Journal of Nursing Research, 33*(1), 63–78.

Hastings-Tolsma, M. 2006. Toward a theory of diversity of human field pattern. *Visions: The Journal of Rogerian Nursing Science, 14*(2): 34–47.

Im, E., W. Chee, E. Guevara, Y. Liu, H. J. Lim, H. M. Tsai et al. 2007. Gender and ethnic differences in cancer pain experience: a multiethnic survey in the united states. *Nursing Research, 56*(5): 296–306.

Kleiber, C., M. Suwanraj, L. Dolan, M. Berg, and A. Kleese. 2007. Pain-sensitive temperament and postoperative pain. *Journal for Specialists in Pediatric Nursing, 12*(3): 149–158.

Langford, R. 2001. *Navigating the maze of nursing research.* St. Louis, MO: Mosby.

Lawrence Berkeley National Laboratory's ELSI Project. 2007. Basic vs applied research revised. Posted to http://*www.lbl.gov/Education/ELSI/research-main.html*

Martin, M. A., M. U. Shalowitz, T. Mijanovich, E. Clark-Kauffman, E. Perez, and C.A. Berry. 2007. The effects of acculturation on asthma burden in a community sample of Mexican-American school children. *American Journal of Public Health, 97*(7): 1290 1296.

McCullagh, M., D. Ronis, and S. Lusk. 2010. Predictors of use of hearing protection among a representative sample of farmers. *Research in Nursing & Health, 33*(6): 528–38.

Miller, J., Y. Guo, and S. Rodseth. 2011. Cluster analysis of intake, output, and voiding habits collected from diary data, *Nursing Research, 60*(2): 115–123.

Nyamathi, A., P. Nahid, J. Berg, J. Burrage, A. Christani, S. Aqtash, D. Morisky, and B. Leake. 2007. Efficacy of Nurse case-managed intervention for latent tuberculosis among homeless subsamples. *Nursing Research, 57*(1): 33–39.

Olbrys, K. 2011. Effect of patient education on post colposcopy follow-up. *Clinical Nursing Research, 20*(2): 209–220.

Olsson, L., J. Karlsson, and I. Ekman. 2007. Effects of nursing interventions within an integrated care pathway for patients with hip fracture. *Journal of Advanced Nursing, 58*(2): 116–125.

Weinert, C., S. Cudney, B. Comstock, and A. Bansal. 2011. Computer intervention impact on psychosocial adaptation of rural women with chronic conditions. *Nursing Research, 60*(2): 82–91.

Yoo, H., S. Kim, H. Hur, and H. Kim. 2011. The effects of an animation distraction intervention on pain response of preschool children during venipuncture. *Applied Nursing Research, (24)*2: 94–100.

Qualitative Research Approaches

CHAPTER OBJECTIVES

1. Describe the purpose of gathering data using qualitative research techniques.
2. Discuss the phases and steps of the qualitative research process.
3. Discuss characteristics of rigor in qualitative research.
4. Identify ethical issues associated with conducting qualitative research.
5. Describe common methods of collecting qualitative data including interviewing, observation, and recording of field notes.
6. Describe commonly used strategies for analyzing qualitative data.
7. Compare and contrast types of qualitative research studies including phenomenology, ethnography, and grounded theory as well as historical study and case studies.

KEY TERMS

Case study research (**p. 151**)

Confirmability (**p. 139**)

Constant comparison (**p. 150**)

Credibility (**p. 139**)

Dependability (**p. 139**)

Ethnography (**p. 147**)

Field (**p. 135**)

Field notes (**p. 141**)

Focus group (**p. 137**)

Grounded theory (**p. 148**)

Hermeneutics (**p. 133**)

Historical research (**p. 150**)

Memo (**p. 142**)

Observation (**p. 137**)

Participants (**p. 135**)

Phenomenology (**p. 133**)

Post-modern existential theory (**p. 134**)

Purposeful sampling (**p. 136**)

Rigor (**p. 138**)

Saturation (**p. 142**)

Semi-structured interview (**p. 137**)

Symbolic interactionism (**p. 133**)

Theoretical sampling (**p. 150**)

Transferability (**p. 139**)

Trustworthiness (**p. 138**)

ABSTRACT

Qualitative research looks and feels very different than quantitative research. This chapter examines how the five phases of the research process apply to qualitative research. It presents three types of qualitative research commonly found in nursing: phenomenology, grounded theory, and ethnography. Additionally, the chapter considers historical research and case study which both use narrative materials for analysis. While qualitative research types have distinct purposes, many of their data collection techniques, such as use of semi-structured interviews and observation, are overlapping. Because narrative data are gathered through interviews, observation, and examination of documents or artifacts, the process of data analysis can be complex and time intensive. Good qualitative researchers will build in processes for data collection and analysis that will strengthen their studies.

This chapter will apply the five phases of the research process to qualitative research. Qualitative research involves systematically collecting, analyzing, and interpreting narrative information. As we saw in Chapter 4, qualitative research differs greatly from traditional quantitative research. It uses an inductive process of discovery that moves from specific cases to broader descriptions of phenomenon. This process provides a depth of understanding not possible in quantitative research. We begin this chapter by presenting an overview of how qualitative researchers implement the phases of the research process. We then describe the types of qualitative research.

The Qualitative Research Process

Chapter 3 introduced the five phases of the research process as a systematic process for gathering information. Chapter 5 applied the five phases to the quantitative research process. Now we will see how these phases also apply to the qualitative process. Figure 7-1 illustrates the phases and steps in the qualitative research process. Note that some of the steps look similar to those in the quantitative process while others are different. The overview discusses each phase of qualitative research and gives examples from a nursing research article.

Phase 1: Conceptualize the Problem

The problem conceptualization phase has four steps. First, the researcher formulates the problem, identifying the area of research concern or interest. Second, he or she moves to the literature to discover further information. Third, the researcher develops the research

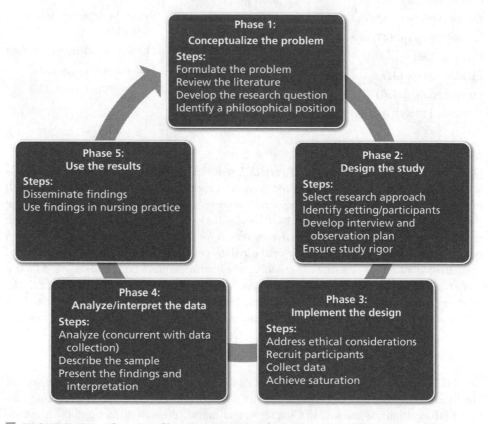

FIGURE 7-1 The Qualitative Research Process
(Adapted from Langford 2001)
Compare Figure 7-1, The Qualitative Research Process to Figure 5-1, The Quantitative Research Process. While the process remains the same, steps are adapted to fit the specific research model.

question. Finally, identifying a philosophic position helps guide the design of the remainder of the study.

FORMULATE THE PROBLEM. In some ways, the initial step in problem conceptualization is actually quite similar to identifying a problem of concern in quantitative research. The concern may arise from a clinical issue or phenomena about which the investigator wished to know more. As in quantitative research, issues arise from practice concerns or lack of information in the literature. Sometimes there may be quantitative studies in the literature, but they may lack the depth or breadth that qualitative studies can provide.

Just as in quantitative studies, qualitative studies discuss the problem statement in one or two paragraphs at the beginning of the article. Background information indicates why the problem merits study and culminates in the statement of the study's purpose. Purpose statements may begin with phrases such as *the purpose of this study is* or be stated in the form of objectives. Identifying a research problem helps the researcher determine which research approach is best. If in-depth discovery and description is a goal, then taking a qualitative approach may be the best fit. The research question is also important in choosing a particular type of qualitative research, explained later in the chapter. Most importantly, a statement of the problem and purpose also provide the reader with key information about the study.

This chapter presents examples of each phase of the research process derived from a published study. Box 7-1 shows a study's problem statement and purpose. Note that the focus of the problem is to examine the everyday lives of the poor who are living with cancer. It tells us that the need for the study is twofold: 1) the poor are more severely affected by cancer and 2) few accounts of their experiences have been documented in the literature. The purpose statement precisely defines the focus of the study. In this case, the study was conducted to better understand the meaning of dignity in the urban poor and

---

BOX 7-1   Sample Problem Statement and Purpose

Hughes, A., M. Gudmundsdottir, and B. Davies. 2007. Everyday struggling to survive: Experiences of the urban poor living with advanced cancer. *Oncology Nursing Forum*, *34*(6): 1113–1118.

Problem Statement

"Vulnerable populations such as the urban poor are disproportionately affected by cancer. The poor face barriers accessing high-quality cancer care and frequently experience insensitivity to their plight. . . . The National Cancer Institute concluded that poor individuals, regardless of race and ethnicity, are diagnosed with more advanced cancer and have lower survival rates than those living in more affluent communities (Singh, Miller, Hankey, and Edwards 2003). That disparity is evident even after controlling for the stage of disease at diagnosis (Singh et al. 2003). Poor people are more likely to die of cancer. Few accounts appear in the literature about the everyday lives of the poor living with advanced cancer and the psychosocial and existential consequences of illness and treatment (Hughes 2005, 2006; Moller 2004; Williams 2004)." (pp. 1113–1114)

Purpose

"Purpose/Objectives: To understand the meaning of dignity to the urban poor and to describe their experiences living with advanced cancer." (p. 1113)

to describe their experiences with cancer. This statement lets the reader know that the participants will be poor people from urban areas with a diagnosis of cancer. Readers also know that not only will the study examine people's experiences with cancer, but will also explore the meaning of dignity.

REVIEW THE LITERATURE. Just as in quantitative research, reviewing the literature is a part of qualitative research. In some instances, literature reviews occur at two points in qualitative studies. At the beginning of the study, a literature review provides essential foundational knowledge about the problem of concern. Literature review is also important at the end of the study, particularly if the investigation uncovered unexpected information related to the study topic. Since the finding was new and unexpected, the researcher may need to go back to the literature to discover more about the unanticipated finding. You may want to review Chapter 2, which focuses on the systematic process of discovering and using information in research.

A concern in qualitative research is that reviewing the literature before a qualitative study begins may bias the researcher's investigation. However, it is important for researchers to know the type of information available on the problem area. Therefore, literature review before the study is an important step. It can prevent unintentional duplication of work and it allows shaping the study to extend knowledge in the field. For example, one reason Hughes et al. (2007) identified for studying the urban poor with cancer, was the limited amount of literature that discussed cancer experiences of this group (see Box 7-1). With this said, researchers should still remain open to unexpected discovery and engage in further literature at the end of the research process.

DEVELOP THE RESEARCH QUESTION. Research questions rather than hypotheses help guide qualitative research. As we saw in Chapter 5, the wording of a hypothesis reflects an if/then prediction: *if* a researcher introduces a particular intervention *x*, *then* the outcome should be *y*. Qualitative research studies occur in less structured settings. Researchers try not to disturb the natural context of the setting (Speziale and Carpenter 2007). They pay of lot of attention to describing what occurs and how it happens. Consequently, qualitative research questions look different from quantitative ones.

Qualitative researchers state questions for investigation in a number of different ways because questions arise from inquiry that is descriptive in nature. They reflect the broader concern of the research exploration and help to focus the research problem. These questions do not contain the independent and dependent variables found in quantitative research. Research questions are broad, open-ended, and non-directional (Creswell 2007). There may be a central over-arching question followed by sub-questions that delineate areas of exploration. Although the Hughes et al. (2007) article did not explicitly state a research question, their study essentially asked "What is the meaning of dignity for the urban poor with advanced cancer?" Additional sub-questions would be "What are the everyday experiences of the urban poor living with advanced cancer?" and "How do the urban poor living with advanced cancer experience dignity?"

IDENTIFY A PHILOSOPHICAL POSITION. As we saw in Chapter 5, researchers use a theoretical framework to identify their research variables and structure the study design. Qualitative research uses theory in a somewhat different way. In qualitative research, a set of assumptions or beliefs called a philosophical orientation or philosophical underpinnings drives the investigative process. Philosophical beliefs underlie different types of qualitative research and infuse the manner in which researchers approach the study. These beliefs influence framing of the research question, choice of method, views about credibility of participants, analysis, and interpretation.

Consider, for example, the philosophical underpinnings of phenomenology. Often, people use the word *phenomenology* without recognizing that it means two things. The term **phenomenology** represents both a set of philosophical beliefs and a specific research methodology. The philosophy of phenomenology can be divided into two broad branches: descriptive phenomenology and hermeneutics (sometimes called interpretive phenomenology). Husserl (1932, 1962) developed early descriptive phenomenological theory. Husserl expressed key ideas about truth and science, including the assertion that the way humans perceive experiences has value and should be studied. Often humans go about their everyday living without critically analyzing their everyday experiences. Research provides a mechanism for learning about lived experiences (Lopez and Willis 2004). Husserl was concerned with objectivity in science. He proposed that in order to avoid bias, researchers must bracket off (shut away) their preconceived ideas and approach the research setting ready to grasp the new information about participants' experiences of their everyday lives.

Martin Heidegger, one of Husserl's students, further advanced philosophical thoughts about phenomenology. His philosophical underpinnings are referred to as either hermeneutic or interpretive phenomenology. **Hermeneutics** deals with the concept of interpretation of text that includes not only writings, but also encompasses interpretation of dialogue and actions (Kvale and Brinkmann 2009). In interpretive phenomenology, Heidegger (1927, 1962) proposed the concept of a *lifeworld* in which the world around individuals intertwines and influences their lives. His concept, called *situated freedom,* asserts that while individuals are free to make some life decisions, their life choices are always influenced by the constraints of the world around them (Lopez and Willis 2004). This idea is different from the one proposed by Husserl, who proposed a radical autonomy free of those constraints. Heidegger also felt that researchers could not bracket their thoughts from the world around them. Researchers were simply too embedded in the world to accomplish bracketing. Instead, Heidegger proposed that researchers benefited from their current knowledge and would use that knowledge when analyzing and interpreting information discovered in the research process. This new knowledge modifies how the researcher thinks about the topic under study and guides further discovery and interpretation.

Consider This . . .

Can scientists mentally bracket off what they already know in order to get a fresh look at the topic under study? What are the research implications of your response?

Another philosophical orientation, **symbolic interactionism**, underlies grounded theory studies and plays a role in how ethnographers think about research as well. Symbolic interactionism recognizes that humans have the capacity to interact with one another and themselves and to derive meaning from those interactions (Blumer 1969). Humans interact with symbols that include physical objects, other humans, language, institutions, ideals, or situations. Meanings are derived out of interactions with objects. For instance, what meaning would a patient derive from a nurse wearing scrubs in a hospital setting or a doctor wearing a white jacket? What types of meanings do these manners of dress have? Nonverbal expressions also send messages. Think about talking to someone who has their arms folded across their chest or yawns during the conversation. What messages do these actions send? Because symbols such as these have meanings for individuals, they make a difference in how people respond to life situations. In studies using symbolic interaction as a philosophical underpinning, the focus is on examining social processes and determining how important symbols influence the world of those individuals.

Consider This . . .

What kinds of objects are important in your world? Do you think being able to explain how these objects play a role in your interactions would help someone else understand more about your world? How so?

Post-modern existential theory forms a basis for some ethnographic research. This theoretical perspective posits that human are unique beings within the context of society and are involved in social change (Manning 1973). The situations in which humans exist are complex and multifaceted, yet often taken for granted in everyday life. Feelings play as important a role as reasoning in determining how individuals respond to their everyday worlds. Approaching research from this perspective helps direct studies toward understanding the everyday life of individuals from their viewpoint. In order to discover the truths of everyday life, the researcher must become part of that world (Manning 1973).

So, how do philosophical underpinnings make a difference in research methods? If one were to use Husserl's philosophical orientation, the researcher would be very concerned about bracketing preconceived ideas during the data collection and analysis process. Researchers might be concerned about relying too much on literature review. If one were to use the interpretive phenomenological approach proposed by Heidegger, researchers would embrace ideas brought to the research field and actively use them to guide the research process.

Box 7-2 shows how Hughes et al. (2007) used an interpretive phenomenological framework. The researchers clearly state their interest in the "concerns, habits, and practices" of their research participants. The researchers proposed using clinical narratives for drawing out those areas since they always contained information about the context in which they occurred.

BOX 7-2 Example of Philosophical Underpinnings

"Interpretive phenomenology served as philosophical background and analytic methodology for this clinical ethnography. . . . Interpretive phenomenology seeks to understand, rather than explain or predict, participants' worlds—their concerns, habits, and practices as they are revealed in narratives; interpretive accounts are always contextualized (Benner 1994). Clinical narratives uncover the practical know-how of symptom recognition and management, help-seeking patterns, and self-care practices for those living with a chronic illness or who are recovering from an injury or illness . . ." (Hughes et al. 2007, p. 1114)

Phase 2: Design the Study

The second phase represents an important step in the planning process because it is when the researcher determines which methods would work best for conducting the investigation. During this phase, researchers make decisions about the study setting, who the participants will be, and how information will be gathered. Four major steps compose this phase: selecting the research approach, identifying the setting and participants, developing the interview plan, and ensuring study rigor.

SELECT A RESEARCH APPROACH. Recall that one of the steps of the first phase was to identify a philosophic position. Since philosophical underpinnings tie to research methodologies, much of the task of selecting a methodology is essentially accomplished before the second step is reached. The research approach guides the focus of the study and key features of data collection and analysis (we discuss the major methods of qualitative research—phenomenology, ethnography, and grounded theory—in greater depth later in this chapter). An important consideration when reading research articles is that rather than identifying a specific method, authors sometimes simply classify their study as a qualitative study. When you see such a broad classification, you need to pay careful attention to the study methods in order to understand the process.

IDENTIFY SETTING AND PARTICIPANTS. To conduct qualitative research, researchers must first identify a setting where potential participants with their "expert knowledge" are available. In qualitative research, the term used to describe a research setting is the **field**. Conducting research in the field is helpful in order to keep participants in a more natural setting where phenomena under study occur. If a researcher wanted to learn more about interactions in an electronic Intensive Care Unit (cICU) where cameras and monitors in an ICU send information to a remote site (the eICU) for further health care provider evaluation, then they would need to talk with nurses and physicians and clerks working in the eICU and do observation in that area. If an investigator wanted to know more about how children managed living in a homeless shelter, then gathering information at the homeless shelter is important.

Once the investigator has identified the field of study, concern turns to strategies for selecting study participants. **Participants** are individuals possessing knowledge about the topic that the researcher wishes to study and who agree to be a part of the research. Sampling in qualitative research has some distinct differences from methods used in quantitative research. First, qualitative researchers use the word *participant* rather than *subject*. This term better reflects the belief that individuals in qualitative studies are not acted upon but rather are active participants in sharing their knowledge about the area of study (Speziale and Carpenter 2007). Remember, participants are the experts in the study. Because of the depth of information gathered, qualitative samples are usually much smaller than those used in quantitative studies. Oftentimes, samples sizes have approximately twenty participants, sometimes more and sometimes less.

Methods used for selecting research participants differ between quantitative and qualitative research. In quantitative research, investigators use random processes to select representative samples in order to generalize findings to other similar groups. Because high study control and generalizability are not the goal, random sampling lacks usefulness in qualitative approaches. However, when investigators are searching for participants who know about the phenomenon of interest, they do not simply choose someone who is conveniently available. Rather, researchers select individuals identified as specifically knowing about or experiencing the phenomenon of interest. For example, a researcher studying eating experiences of adolescents undergoing bone marrow transplants would need to talk with those adolescents (Rodgers, Young, Hockenberry, Binder, and Symes 2010). Interviewing parents of those adolescents might not reveal the same concerns.

A term commonly used to describe the sampling process in qualitative research is purposeful (or purposive) sampling. In **purposeful sampling**, researchers select participants because of their first-hand knowledge about the phenomenon. For example, if researchers want to know about how frail elderly women manage living independently in their own homes, then they must talk with elderly women who are independently managing. Oftentimes, as researchers analyze data during the study, they may identify information gaps and search for individuals with specific characteristics that can fill that gap. For example, in a study on nursing job satisfaction, investigators might discover that they need additional male participants or more nurses who are new to the profession. This consideration would influence the selection of the next potential participant.

When investigators initiate a study, they may not always know whom all of their participants may be or where they will find them, particularly if potential participants are difficult to locate. To facilitate data collection, investigators use a sampling technique called snowballing or network sampling. In this method, the researcher asks a participant enrolled in the study if they might know of other individuals that are knowledgeable about the study topic. The investigator would then contact that individual. For example, when Gaudine, LeFort, Lamb, and Thorne (2011) studied clinical ethical conflicts of nurses and physicians, they initially identified nurses, nurse managers, and physicians to interview. As researchers, they were unaware of all nurses and physicians experiencing ethical conflicts. At the time of the interview, researchers asked participants to identify other potential contacts who were subsequently approached for study participation.

Box 7-3 discusses the identification and selection of participants for Hughes et al. (2007) study of urban poor living with cancer. Note the participants' first-hand knowledge of being poor and living with cancer. Rather than using the snowballing technique discussed above, researchers enlisted the aid of other health care providers who were knowledgeable about participant characteristics that would make them suitable for study participation. Over the course of a qualitative study, researchers consistently communicate with other health care providers who can help to identify potential participants. This process permits selection of participants with specific characteristics that have the potential to fill in gaps in the study analysis.

DEVELOP INTERVIEW AND OBSERVATION PLAN. Investigators employ several data collection techniques to gather information in qualitative studies. While interviewing is the most commonly used technique, observation may play a role in data collection as well.

BOX 7-3   Example of Study Setting and Participants

"Participants were recruited from providers caring for the urban poor including an oncology clinic in a public hospital, case managers, and home health care clinicians and other social service providers working with the poor. Participants were eligible for the study if they were 18 years of age or older, able to speak and understand English, able to provide informed consent, poor, diagnosed with advanced cancer, and aware of the seriousness of their illness" (Hughes et al. 2007, p. 1114).

Interviewing represents a pragmatic way of gathering information about a diverse array of topics. Kvale and Brinkmann (2009) suggest that "if you want to know how people understand their world and their life, why not talk with them?" (p. *xvii*) Indeed, interviews may have a somewhat conversational nature and do provide a way to get substantial amounts of information quickly. **Semi-structured interviews**, usually guided by a short series of broad open-ended questions, allow exploration of peoples' experiences or understandings regarding the area of study. Open-ended questions permit individual variation in responses and participants are able to express how they understand or experience a particular situation. Researchers sometimes use sub-questions or probes to elicit further information. Audio-recording interviews helps to preserve the nature and context of the information. Once interviews are completed, researchers often transcribe the recordings verbatim and subsequently use them for analysis. One step taken to ensure confidentiality is that any names or other personal identifiers that might have occurred on the tape would be removed. Sometimes an alternate name for a person or place called a pseudonym is substituted.

The **focus group** is a close cousin to the semi-structured interview, except that rather than individual interviews, small groups of about six to eight participants come together and respond to open-ended questions regarding a selected area. A study may have one or several focus groups or focus groups may be combined with individual interviews. One advantage of this method is that group synergy can spur individuals to recall incidents or memories related to the research topic. A disadvantage is that participants may not share important information in a group setting that they might have divulged in an individual interview. Focus groups are usually audio-recorded and the recordings are transcribed word for word and analyzed.

Sometimes researchers observe study participants in the social situation of their world rather than relying only on information shared in interviews. **Observation** has its roots in anthropology and is an important part of ethnographic studies, although phenomenological and grounded theory studies may incorporate this information-gathering technique as well. Advantages of incorporating observation into a study are that investigators (a) have direct access to reality and (b) can discover if information participants have shared matches what is happening. Observation may also help investigators discover and explore relevant areas that interviews had not previously revealed. This discovery can help researchers to ask relevant interview questions and gain a better understanding of the social context. Recording data during observation requires careful planning. Field notes and memos, devices discussed later in this chapter, facilitate documentation of observational events.

Observation requires the presence of the researcher in the research setting. When doing observation, researchers must decide what to observe. Researchers may have a specific agenda for observation or may want to examine how things unfold in the natural setting. There are two modalities for observation: *non-participant* and *participant observation*. In non-participant observation, the investigator simply watches individuals in a natural research setting. In an ethnographic study of an eICU, the researcher may go to the unit, sit in an unobtrusive area, and observe what is happening while business is conducted as usual (Stafford, Meyers, Young, Foster, and Huber 2008). Although the researcher is present, she/he does not play any other role in the unit. In participant observation, the researcher actually has a role in the setting while they are collecting information for the study. For example, in an ethnographic study of an AIDS hospice, one of the investigators also worked as a volunteer for the hospice during the study (Kotarba and Hurt 1995). Observation brings up special ethical issues. It is important for individuals to know that a research study is in progress and for them to consent to be a part of that process. Logistically, securing consent for observation from all those present in the setting is difficult.

> **Consider This . . .**
>
> If you were a participant in a qualitative study, in what ways might your behavior differ if you knew you were being observed?

When using semi-structured interviewing and observation as data collection techniques, researchers engage participants in ways where information sharing is quite personal. Researchers, perhaps especially nurses, need to remind themselves that they are working in a researcher mode and that their function is to gather information. In the researcher role, investigators should avoid slipping into a nursing role. It is easier to maintain the research role by clearly defining the study purpose and the role of the researcher. When engagement for data collection consists of more than one visit or interview, at the beginning of each session researchers can remind participants about the purpose and the researcher's role. If participants need nursing care or other forms of care, then the researcher should make the appropriate referrals.

Documents and other records also play a role in qualitative data collection (Patton 2002). Operation manuals, institutional descriptions or web sites, minutes from meetings, logs, or other records may contain information that further describes context and operations of the study setting. Written narratives and/or reflective journaling from research participants provide useful information because participants have time to reflect about the information shared (Speziale and Carpenter 2007). Photos and video-taping also provide rich data resources for analysis.

Today's high technology world allows generation of data through asynchronous and synchronous online formats. In a nursing education research study, investigators used the social media Facebook to locate previously enrolled nursing students for study participation (Amerson 2010). Asynchronous online discussions have provided text used for analysis in qualitative study (Hew and Cheung 2008). When studying breast-feeding practices of mothers who had experienced traumatic births, Beck and Watson (2008) used the Internet to recruit participants, who then sent their narratives on breast-feeding experiences to the investigators. Blogs also provide sources of narrative information. With the advent and use of new technologies for gathering data, researchers must carefully proceed in order to uphold the ethical principles of research (Heilferty 2011; Kennedy 2008). One particular consideration is whether information is in the public domain or private domain. Ethically sound research practices must consider issues of consent, confidentiality, and privacy as technology moves ahead (Heilferty 2011; Kennedy 2008).

ENSURE STUDY RIGOR. Maintaining rigor in the research process is an important consideration that begins with planning the study and continues through implementation and analysis. Scientific **rigor** means that studies are conducted such that professionals who wish to use the research findings will be assured of the quality. **Trustworthiness** is a term denoting scientific rigor in qualitative research. Trustworthiness consists of four concerns that research studies should address in their planning, implementation, and analysis: credibility, transferability, dependability, and confirmability (Lincoln and Guba 1985). It is important to think about how to incorporate these aspects during the study planning process. **Credibility** refers to the truthfulness or believability of the findings. One way to ensure credibility is to have extended contact with participants in the field. A technique called *member checking*, in which investigators return to the field and talk to participants about the emerging findings, can ascertain if participants think findings are accurate (Speziale and Carpenter 2007). **Transferability** refers to the ability to transfer study findings to other similar situations. We have already stated that generalizability is not the goal of qualitative studies. However, researchers should provide sufficient information about the context of the study to facilitate decisions made by others about the usability of the information in their settings. **Dependability** examines how stable or constant qualitative data remain over time. Since data collection and analysis are concurrent processes, the researcher's understanding of a phenomenon shifts as the research continues. This shift leads to changes in sampling strategies and identification of additional interview questions or new areas to probe. Investigators must thoroughly describe data collection methods, noting adaptations made while in the field, as well as analytic processes (Speziale and Carpenter 2007). Finally, **confirmability** captures a sense of objectivity in the research. The question of confirmability is "Would others examining these data confirm the findings?" Audit trails are an accounting of the research process that provides a record of analytic decision-making others can track. Throughout the study process, investigators keep notes regarding the methods used for data collection and analytic decisions. This process permits another researcher to review the analysis to see if their interpretation of the findings is similar to that of the original investigators (Speziale and Carpenter 2007). Box 7-4 presents an example of a discussion regarding study rigor that appeared in the Hughes et al. (2007) study about the urban poor living with cancer. Note the strategies used such as the prolonged participant contact, debriefing, in-depth description, and member checking.

Phase 3: Implement the Design

After all of the work conceptualizing and planning the study, implementing the study design represents an exciting phase. This phase includes four key steps: addressing ethical considerations, recruiting participants, collecting data, and achieving saturation.

ADDRESS ETHICAL CONSIDERATIONS. Chapter 4 presented basic information about ethical considerations of research. Just as in quantitative research, qualitative studies must have an institutional review board (IRB) approval and participants must give informed consent

---

BOX 7-4   Example of Use of Rigor

"The data collection procedures and resulting interpretive accounts were monitored carefully throughout the study to ensure scientific rigor. Strategies to promote rigor included prolonged and persistent field observations to build trust and appreciate cultural nuances, debriefing by the principal investigator (PI) with the research team to review observations and impressions, comparing and contrasting the interpretations of the data, recognizing the researcher's position that may have influenced what was unseen and unheard, providing rich and thick descriptions for readers to verify the trustworthiness of the claims, and member checks with participants about preliminary impressions . . ." (Hughes et al. 2007, p. 1114).

prior to the study. In addition to the usual protections afforded research participants, special consideration in qualitative research relates to confidentiality, the relationship of researcher to participant, and the sensitivity of the issues discussed.

Confidentially is of particular concern in qualitative research because the use of recording devices such as audio-taping, and in some instances video-taping, provide an identification trail that potentially can lead back to participants (Speziale and Carpenter 2007). Research consents must clearly explain the risk of potential loss of confidentiality. Protection of confidentiality is achieved by limiting the persons who have access to taped materials and securing these materials in locked files or password protected computers. Participants in qualitative studies are almost never anonymous. Data collection techniques using voice recordings or participant observation mean that at the very least, investigators know the participant's identity. Lack of research participant anonymity provides a strong impetus for investigators to ensure confidentiality. Following research completion, destruction of original taped materials or audio files destroys linking information. Another issue related to confidentiality is that examples and stories about the phenomenon under study may contain identifying information. However, changing participants' names, locations, or other key identifiable data can protect their identities (Patton 2002). For example, renaming a hospital where a patient is located to something generic such as "Mercy Hospital" protects identities of participants from those reading the published research.

Interviews and observation in qualitative research involve sharing information, which potentially allows for formation of a relationship between researcher and participant that is not part of the research purpose. Personal stories and dialogs about sensitive topics and prolonged engagement consisting of multiple interviews or observations may permit the formation of a relationship or end with a therapeutic effect for the participant that is outside of the research goal (Eide and Kahn 2008). While therapeutic effects are not a promised outcome of research participation, the researcher is often the first person who has asked about particular participant experiences. Researchers examining qualitative research ethics report that participants describe the opportunity to share their story as a benefit when facing a chronic diagnosis (Townsend, Cox, and Li 2010). Participants sometimes find a sense of relief when they share their story. Prior to the study, researchers should clearly identify the purpose of the research and their role of researcher, not counselor (Speziale and Carpenter 2007). Additionally, if there is prolonged engagement with study participants and settings over an extended time period, researchers should create a plan for gracefully withdrawing from the study setting (Lofland, Snow, Anderson, and Lofland 2006). For example, researchers need to let participants know when the study is ending. Researchers may need a formal goodbye to participants. If reports of study findings were promised, researchers should honor those promises.

Finally, the topic of research may be a sensitive one that will evoke emotions in persons interviewed. For example, McGahey-Oakland, Lieder, Young, and Jefferson (2007) interviewed parents of pediatric patients who had undergone cardio-pulmonary resuscitation about their experiences. Because several of the children had died during the resuscitation attempt, the topic was quite sensitive. Prior to conducting the study, researchers needed to give the IRB sufficient justification regarding benefits of having the information gathered. Special considerations during the interview included preparation for crying, stopping interviews either at the request of the participant or discretion of the investigator, and availability of counseling or other support resources for participants, if needed.

RECRUIT PARTICIPANTS. As we said in our discussion of Phase 2, study design identifies the research setting and potential participant characteristics. A key to successfully conducting a qualitative study is identifying and obtaining access to the research field. Access occurs on two levels: *formal access* and *informal access*. Formal access occurs when researchers need to obtain institutional permission in order to conduct research in a setting. For example, if the research were to occur in a hospital, clinic, or community agency, the researchers must obtain formal approval. They may need to show the institution

a. the reason they want use that institution for the study,

b. what will be done during the study,

c. if study participation would cause disruption to routines, and

d. what will be gained from the study—both by the participants and information that might be useful to the institution.

Informal access includes two aspects that can directly affect participant recruitment. First, potential participants must be willing to sign the informed consent for study participation and actually allow themselves to be observed and/or participate in the interview. Second, some field studies may have informal group leaders or "gatekeepers" that need to sanction the presence of a researcher and give group members the option to participate. This issue is particularly important in ethnographic studies where group dynamics are an important part of the study. Even with official permission, it is important to identify informal gatekeepers. When the informal gatekeeper indicates that the investigator is OK to work with, it enhances their access to potential participants willing to take part in the study.

COLLECT DATA. During the design phase, researchers develop a semi-structured interview guide. As participants are recruited, audio-taped interviews are conducted using the interview guide. Researchers must be attentive in order to guide the interview process and use probing questions to gain greater depth of information or explore new areas uncovered during the interview. As the study progresses and new information emerges, changes may take place in the questions used on the interview schedule. Researchers may find that there are additional areas that need exploration and develop new questions. They may discover that some questions lose their relevance as the study continues. Observation offers the opportunity to corroborate information heard in interviews. It may also identify new areas that interviews need to address.

Researchers use field notes and memos to record information associated with the data collection and analysis process. Often the use of **field notes** is specifically associated with ethnographic studies and refers to the written comments that investigators make during the process of observation. Field notes may be made during or immediately after the observation process and consist of recording any information about the context of the situation being observed, of specific behaviors or activities observed, or of notes about impressions or thoughts regarding the observations (Speziale and Carpenter 2007). For example, when observing health care providers working in an eICU, a researcher's field notes included a drawing of the layout of the eICU room and the position of different care providers (Stafford et al. 2008). Other field notes included information about the technology connecting the eICU to the actual ICU, worker attire, conversations, method used for rounding on ICU patients, and interventions in an emergency.

Memos serve a function similar to field notes. **Memos** are simply a method of systematic record-keeping about analytical decision-making that occurs throughout the study. They provide a mechanism for recording researcher reflections from the inception of the study through the analysis (Birks, Chapman, and Francis 2008). For example, as the study begins, memos may discuss how decisions were made to select research participants. After interviews are begun, memos provide a way to record researcher thinking about the information obtained. Memos can provide a snapshot of the researcher's thinking at a particular phase of the study (Birks et al. 2008, p. 71).

Box 7-5 provides an example of the data collection process reported in the urban poor living with cancer study (Hughes et al. 2007). Notice how researchers kept field notes regarding their observations. Not only did patients participate in the study, but informal interviews were also conducted with the health and social service providers to add context and perspective to the information gathered.

ACHIEVE SATURATION. As noted previously, qualitative studies tend to have smaller sample sizes than quantitative studies. One criteria used for determining sample size is the concept of saturation. **Saturation** occurs when the researcher is no longer hearing new information from research participants that adds to understanding of the phenomenon (Creswell 2007). When researchers begin to hear the same explanations related to the study topic repeatedly, they know they have achieved saturation. Saturation also happens when participants begin to confirm previously collected data. When researchers no longer learn anything new from interviews, they conclude that the data are saturated and that it is time to end data collection.

Phase 4: Analyze and Interpret the Data

Analysis of qualitative data is somewhat different in nature from quantitative analysis. One unusual feature of data analysis is that the process begins when the first data are collected. Steps in this phase include analyzing the data, describing the sample, and presenting the findings.

ANALYZE DATA. Data analysis begins with the first interview. Generally, data analysis consists of transcribing the audio-taped data and field notes into typed transcripts. While some investigators type their own tape transcriptions, others send them to a transcription

---

BOX 7-5   Example Data Collection

"Interview transcripts and field notes provided the primary qualitative data for the analysis. Informal interviews of health and social service providers working with the study population and observations regarding environments where patients lived or received care were recorded in the field notes. Fourteen patients were interviewed as many as three times, for a total of 32 interviews; two patients with advanced cancer who were domestic partners asked to be interviewed as a couple. Interviews were conducted wherever convenient for participants: single-room occupancy hotels, housing projects, and other residences, hospital rooms, coffee shops, a residential hospice, or building lobbies. Participants were asked to describe their experiences living with cancer, provide narratives of interactions with health care providers, and discuss what dignity meant to them. Data were collected from January 2006 through January 2007" (Hughes et al. 2007, p. 1114).

service if funding is available. Regardless of who completes the transcription, it is a good idea to listen to the audiotape while reading the transcript to ensure accuracy.

Data analysis is a time-consuming and potentially mentally taxing process. Generally, uninterrupted time periods facilitate the analysis process because it allows researchers the ability to maintain their train of thought. Each of the qualitative methodologies has steps that systematically guide the analysis process. While there are many different processes with steps for data analysis, basic steps include:

- reading and rereading the transcript to obtain a feel for the information that is shared,
- identifying information that tends to cluster together,
- developing a description for themes that emerge, providing an interpretative statement for the theme, and
- supporting the identified theme with evidence.

Steps for analysis are often more proscribed in phenomenological and grounded theory studies and somewhat more fluid in ethnographic studies. Computer programs can facilitate the analysis process by providing a mechanism for data organization. Box 7-6 provides an example of the data analysis process for the urban poor with cancer study. Note the discussion regarding tape transcription, transcript review, comparison across cases, and thematic identification. These steps are common elements of qualitative analysis.

DESCRIBE THE SAMPLE. Even though qualitative studies analyze narrative, sample description may also involve some numerical aspects, although the descriptive statistics may not be as complete or sophisticated as those found in quantitative ones. Sample description provides a context for the study and can help readers determine the information's potential transferability. The sample description in the Hughes study we have been exploring consists of both numeric and narrative analysis (Box 7-7). From this information, readers can derive that the sample was diverse, included both men and women with solid tumors, and represented an age range of 25 years. With that description, others wishing to use the findings may identify how similar the study sample is to the groups of people for whom they care.

BOX 7-6 Example of Data Analysis

"Interviews and field notes were audio-taped and transcribed verbatim and later verified for accuracy. Transcripts were read and reread and interviews were compared and contrasted within and across cases. Identifying paradigm cases is an analytic strategy to begin to understand a test; paradigm cases are 'strong instances of concerns or ways of being in the world' (Benner, 1994, p. 113). Thematic analysis allows cross-case comparisons of distinctions and patterns; not infrequently, the incongruities and inconsistencies of human beings emerge (Benner, 1994). The PI drafted and redrafted interpretive memos of themes and exemplars that were discussed and revised with the research team to develop an interpretive account. All participant names used in this article are pseudonyms" (Hughes et al. 2007, p. 1114).

BOX 7-7   Example of Sample Description

"The sample was racially diverse and reflective of the city's English-speaking population of the urban poor with cancer. Fourteen patients, six men and eight women with Stage III or IV solid tumors participated. The sample ranged in age from 45 to 69 years, and 50% were people of color (five African Americans and two Hispanics or Latinos). Seven patients had a history of homelessness. Of note, seven patients died by the completion of data collection, some within days or weeks of being interviewed" (Hughes et al. 2007, pp. 1114–1115).

PRESENT THE FINDINGS AND INTERPRETATIONS. Many novice readers tend to find qualitative studies easier to follow than quantitative ones because they present their findings in narrative form. Findings should present a comprehensive picture of the phenomenon, description of a cultural group, or of the theory developed. Evidence obtained through interviews and observations should support the findings discussion. Box 7-8 presents an example of some of the findings from the Hughes study. Note how researchers have grouped together the common concerns and perceptions of participants. Although the sample was diverse, commonalities existed that shed light on the experiences of the urban poor living with cancer.

Phase 5: Use the Results

As in quantitative research, the final phase is perhaps the most important. Research studies take time, energy, and resources. In order to make these expenditures worthwhile, findings need to be disseminated and put into practice.

BOX 7-8   Example of Summary of the Findings

"For everyone, rich and poor alike, being diagnosed with cancer occurs in the middle of a life, within the context of pre-existing challenges and possibilities. The urban poor with cancer in this study struggled with concerns about housing, personal safety on dangerous streets and neighborhoods, transportation to appointments, limited money for medication copayments, and healthcare systems where many previously felt unwelcomed and avoided 'unless dying.' Some believed their illness was not taken seriously because they did not have the right insurance; all were dependent on overburdened public healthcare systems or faith-based community clinics for care" (Hughes et al. 2007, p. 1116).

Findings further described the difficult backgrounds of participants even in their younger years—although not all patients were homeless and some continued to work part time. Because patients had cancer diagnoses for several years, most were found to be living with cancer rather than dying. They preferred to think of themselves as survivors and were reluctant to discuss death even though for some it was near. Participants described struggles with the health care system and their providers. An example included being sent alone to a one-room hotel following surgery while still too weak to do self-care.

Researchers concluded "the experience of advanced cancer occurred in the context of lives, that in most cases, were already challenged and wanting. They had been struggling with life; cancer was at times just one more burden to endure" (Hughes et al. 2007, p. 1117).

DISSEMINATE FINDINGS. A critical factor in qualitative research is clearly organizing information and writing up the findings. This step is the most essential portion of the paperwork. The descriptions offered by qualitative research can influence nurses both on a professional and personal level. Describing the collective worlds of study participants can have more of an impact than quantitative studies. Qualitative research offers an opportunity to tell the collective story of groups such as women experiencing intimate partner violence, or of cancer survivors, or of those coping with a chronic illness. It offers an in-depth picture that is difficult to obtain through quantitative studies. Therefore, qualitative researchers should work to produce presentations and manuscripts that accurately portray the research findings.

USE THE FINDINGS. When investigators propose and conduct research studies, they need to be concerned with the "so what?" factor. What about this study and its findings is useful in clinical practice? If findings fail to have an impact on practice, then one has to wonder why conducting the study was so important. This segment will reiterate the message found in Chapter 5: *as consumers of research, nurses must decide how to apply findings in practice*. Look back at the example study of the urban poor living with cancer. As a nurse, do the findings shed light on the cancer experience? Do these findings suggest areas that may need intervention? For example, what should happen with patients who cannot do self-care following surgery? Are there potential ways to relieve some of the burden of dealing with cancer and the other day-to-day burdens these participants described? Qualitative studies can offer insight into the world of health care. Pay attention, learn, and apply.

Types of Qualitative Research

As you have seen in the last two chapters, many different types of study approaches fall under the classification of quantitative research. Qualitative research has several different types of approaches as well. This chapter discusses in depth three of the most common types of qualitative research: phenomenology, ethnography, and grounded theory. A good question to ask is "why are different types of qualitative studies needed?" As you will discover, each type of qualitative research has a different purpose and each produces a different product such as an in-depth description, a theory, or a description of a culture. Two other forms of research that use narrative materials in data collection and analysis are historical research and case study. This chapter discusses these as well.

Phenomenology

A phenomenon is something that is experienced or is the way that someone perceives or understands a particular thing. As such, phenomenological studies try to discover how people make sense of their world. People attempt to master their world by generating practical knowledge about how things work. The way individuals perceive experiences or things depends on the social context and individual interpretation about the meaning of the experience. Although people understand the meanings of experiences or things from an individual perspective, commonalities of experience exist among groups. In order to better understand how people interpret their world, a phenomenological researcher examines the commonalities and differences of peoples' interpretations of their experiences. Typical research questions in phenomenological studies relate to the nature of specific experiences, for example "what are parents' experiences of being present during resuscitation of their child?" or "what are patient experiences of living with their cancer diagnosis?" Box 7-9 summarizes a phenomenological study by Snyder (2006). Investigators studied the experiences of women living with polycystic ovary syndrome. This hormonal disorder increases the blood levels of androgens and increases secretions of insulin. Women no longer ovulate and experience increased facial hair growth, acne, balding, menstrual dysfunction, and infertility (Snyder 2006). The risk for cardiovascular disease and cancer increases. Although not explicitly stated, the research question for this study could be "what is the lived experience of women with polycystic ovary syndrome?"

To learn about the fundamental nature of experience, researchers must go to the individuals who have had that experience to get an in-depth description of it. In this sense, the true experts regarding the research topic are the people who can offer their perspective on a particular experience. In Snyder's (2006) study, open-ended interview questions explored women's experiences and allowed researchers to encourage women to further expand and offer examples to clarify information shared.

During and following intensive interviews with people about the nature and meaning of the experience, the investigator analyzes and interprets the narrative information by identifying and describing common themes from the recorded dialogues. Snyder makes reference to using a systematic analytic process designed by Giorgi. Giorgi's (1985) steps guide investigators through the analytic process by establishing guidelines that

---

BOX 7-9   Sample Summary of a Phenomenological Study

Snyder, B. 2006. The lived experience of women diagnosed with polycystic ovary syndrome. *Journal of Obstetric, Gynecology, and Neonatal Nursing, 35*(3): 385–392.

Snyder (2006) studied the experiences of women diagnosed with polycystic ovary syndrome (PCOS). Using a phenomenological approach, Snyder obtained a purposive sample of 12 premenopausal women previously diagnosed with PCOS. Women in her sample represented a range of ages, race, and time-periods following diagnosis. Audio-taped semi-structured interviews were used to collect data. The investigator transcribed and analyzed the interviews by grouping similar thoughts and experiences into categories.

Analysis began with the first interview transcript and proceeded throughout the data collection process. Snyder systematically compared each of the interviews to all of the other interviews. An analysis method by Giorgi guided the process. Seven themes were identified, including (a) *Identifying differences* in which women with PCOS identified themselves as being different from other women without the syndrome; (b) *Acknowledging impact on femininity* where physical changes such as hair growth and obesity made women feel less feminine; (c) *Searching for answers* because women frequently had difficulty getting answers about what was happening to them; (d) *Wanting to be normal* reflected the women's desires to look and physiologically function more like other women without PCOS; (e) *Gaining control* where women were able to understand what was happening to their bodies and plan their lives around it; (f) *Letting go of guilt* described how women understood that their obesity was related to an underlying disorder rather than a lack of control; and (g) *Dealing with it* where women managed day-to-day uncertainty.

systematically move researchers through the narrative information. There are a number of different systematic processes available to phenomenological researchers to guide analysis. Philosophical underpinnings drive the exact character of the analytic steps. These steps help researchers to organize information into meaningful descriptions of the phenomenon, usually involving identification of themes derived from commonalities of participant descriptions about their experiences. The final product of a phenomenological study is a comprehensive, narrative description that describes and interprets the themes. In Snyder's (2006) study on women living with polycystic ovary syndrome the application goal was to add to the knowledge base about polycystic ovary syndrome and thus enable health care providers to improve health outcomes and well-being of these women. Note the common elements of the experience of living with polycystic ovary syndrome. As you read the themes, ask yourself if this information would assist you as a nurse in relating to women with polycystic ovary syndrome.

Ethnography

Ethnography is a field research tradition that has its roots in anthropology. Classically defined, ethnographies reflect the work of describing a culture (Spradley 1979). It is both a process as well as the end product of the completed study. Researchers conduct ethnographic studies when they want to know more about people and the group of which they are a part. In classical anthropological studies, investigators might go and live with a village to discover how the village worked and observe the life practices in which they engaged. In contemporary ethnography, a group might be composed of a group of patients or health care providers or a combination of patients and health care providers at a particular place. When conducting ethnography, researchers enter into the world of respondents as if they were a stranger. From the stranger's perspective, researchers then attempt to discover how that village works. To conduct an ethnographic study, the investigator needs to be in the field with the group they are studying. Consequently, in addition to interviews, observation plays a key role in the data collection process.

Research questions in ethnography center around everyday life and seek to discover meanings which are taken for granted. For example, Kotarba and Hurt (1995) conducted an ethnography of an AIDS hospice where they talked to health care providers, patients, and families about their experiences and subsequently described the everyday experiences of life in a hospice. Another example is completing an ethnographic study in an eICU department where a group of health care workers working from a room with high technology computers and cameras provide supplemental support to intensive care staff that are actually on the unit (Stafford et al. 2008).

Consider This . . .

If you were a participant observer, what kinds of things would you need to consider in order to gather data while playing a role as a participant? How might this be different if you were a nonparticipant observer?

Box 7-10 provides a summary of an ethnographic study. Examine the ethnographic components of this study. Believing that cultural beliefs influenced understanding of mental illness, investigators were specifically interested in understanding mental health within the community context of recently immigrated Mexican adolescents. This study's

> **BOX 7-10   Sample Summary of an Ethnographic Study**
>
> Garcia, C. and E. Saewyc. 2007. Perceptions of mental health among recently immigrated Mexican adolescents. *Issues in Mental Health Nursing, 28*: 37–54.
>
> Garcia and Saewyc (2007) investigated the perceptions of mental health among 14 Mexican adolescent girls who had recently immigrated to the United States. They conducted an initial interview using a semi-structured guide with open-ended questions focusing on health, influences, and experiences accessing the health care system. During the next phase of the study, the adolescents were given 24-exposure disposable cameras and asked to take pictures of living in the United States. Investigators interviewed the adolescents again after developing the pictures, asking them to share descriptions and the significance of the pictures. In addition, the investigators completed participant observation and kept field notes.
>
> The adolescents described the mental aspect of health within the framework of physical, mental, and social attributes. Mental health encompassed good physical health, a positive attitude and being happy, and positive thinking. Mentally unhealthy individuals had problems from stress and anxiety and poor health habits such as lack of sleep or poor nutrition. Stresses of immigration from fitting in or missing those remaining in Mexico also influenced mental health. Promoting health included talking with friends, families, and occasionally health care providers. Acting as a role model for friends or peers also promoted health. One important finding was that participants were unaware of who they could turn to for mental health problems and did not see health care providers as resources.

aim is congruent with the aims of ethnography. Investigators posited that having a better understanding of cultural beliefs would lead to better services for preventing and treating mental health disorders. Note the data techniques used. Investigators used semi-structured interviews to gather information about health, behaviors, and health care access. To expand cultural understanding, participants took photographs about life and health in the community. Investigators then used the photos in additional interviews to gather information about the perceptions and meanings of health. Finally, participant observation served as a third mechanism to gather information about the environment.

Investigators systematically analyzed information from all of these information sources to explicate a picture of mental health for Mexican adolescents. How usable are these findings? Investigators specifically uncovered facilitators for mental health somewhat unique for this immigrant population. Barriers existed for mental health care access. A chilling finding was that adolescents did not see health care providers as resources. So, the study provided initial insight into mental health perceptions of recently immigrated Mexicans, suggested the need for further research, and provided useful information to guide development of mental health services to this group.

Grounded Theory

In the quantitative research chapters, one of the purposes of research was to take a theory, develop a hypothesis related to tenets of that theory, and then test the hypothesis to determine if the theory was correct. Moving from a general theory to a specific hypothesis is a deductive process. **Grounded theory** works the opposite direction of this method. Rather than beginning with a theory, researchers seek to discover new information that leads to the development of a relevant theory. This process is inductive in that the researcher begins with a specific situation from which a more generalized theory is drawn. The developed theory is the end product.

The goal of grounded theory is to develop useful theories that are relevant to real world phenomena (Glaser and Strauss 1967). In grounded theory research, researchers are working from the ground up because they do not have a preconceived idea about what the research outcome will be. Rather, investigators know the area researched, gather data about that area, and then examine the data to see the kinds of information that emerge. In other words, the resulting theory is grounded in the data from which it was developed. Theories developed are not merely descriptive: rather, researchers tie together the concepts they discover to create an integrated, cohesive theory.

Research questions tend to center around concerns or problems that are important to practice with the goal of developing a theory. For example, "how do sexual assault survivors seek help with emotional recovery (Symes 2000)?" Or, "how do nurses acquire knowledge for giving spiritual care (Hood, Olson, and Allen 2007)?" Box 7-11 describes a grounded theory study conducted by Reb (2007). Through the grounded theory process, she examined hope in women facing ovarian cancer, uncovering phases following diagnosis.

Usually, data are collected via interviews and sometimes observation. Note that in the summary of her article, Reb used semi-structured interviewing to discern the role of

---

BOX 7-11 **Sample Summary of a Grounded Theory Study**

Reb, A. 2007. Transforming the death sentence: Elements of hope in women with advanced ovarian cancer. *Oncology Nursing Forum, 34*(6): E70–E81.

Reb (2007) used a grounded theory approach to discover how women diagnosed with advanced ovarian cancer maintained hope. Twenty women participated in semi-structured interviews about their experiences of diagnosis and treatment. As interviews were conducted, Reb used constant comparison to analyze transcripts as they were obtained, comparing them to earlier transcripts. Women felt they were "facing a death threat" and the core or central variable tied to maintaining hope was "transforming the death sentence" (p. E72). Transforming the death sentence occurred over three phases that included "shock" of initial diagnoses, "aftershock" where they began to grasp reality, and finally "rebuilding" their lives within a new paradigm.

Stages during the shock phase included *sensing the threat* where women sensed something wrong; *succumbing to the vortex* where women felt overwhelmed with the diagnosis, and *surviving the chaos* where women adopted measures to prepare for treatment and to gather (or avoid gathering) additional information (Reb 2007, p. E73). The "aftershock" phase included *acknowledging the fear* of recurrence or dying; *mobilizing resources* as women sought ways to maintain control over the situation; and *internalizing the illness* where women recognized their lives were totally changing (p. E 74). During "rebuilding" women began to live in a new paradigm in which they *managed uncertainty* while trying to get on with their lives; *shifting expectations* as goals were revised and meaningful priorities were selected; and *searching for meaning* where women tried to adopt a new perspective, often focusing on day-to-day living and relationships. Strategies emerged regarding how women increased and maintained situational control through each phase. Spiritual beliefs increased hope.

hope for women diagnosed with a disease with a high mortality rate. Interviewers asked questions such as "what does the word hope mean to you personally?" (p. E71) and traced experiences before and after the ovarian cancer diagnosis.

Grounded theory stresses the discovery and development of theories from data that are systematically gathered and rigorously analyzed (Strauss and Corbin 1998). Data collection and analysis begin almost simultaneously using a technique called **constant comparison** where researchers compare the second transcribed interview to the first; then, the third interview to the first and second ones and so forth. Note that Reb (2007) used constant comparison as part of her systematic analysis. Coding processes help the researcher to identify relevant concepts in a process called open coding, group similar concepts in the axial coding phase, and then examine the interconnectedness of the concepts during selective coding (Strauss and Corbin 1998).

In grounded theory research, **theoretical sampling** identifies specific procedures used for the sampling process that are associated with the coding phase. Very simply, the concept behind theoretical sampling is that as investigators begin to organize and code data to develop their evolving theory, they make a decision about whom to next approach and what questions to ask. In grounded theory, theoretical sampling has three phases:

- *Open sampling*, completed early in the study, enables the investigator to gather as much information as possible about the study topic. The process is very open to persons, places, and events where investigators can uncover the most relevant information about the study topic (Strauss and Corbin 1998).

- During *relational or variational sampling*, researchers are in the phase of the study where they are further developing study categories and subcategories. Rather than taking anyone who might know something about the topic, investigators are looking for individuals who have knowledge that is more specific.

- *Discriminate sampling* occurs during the final phase of a grounded theory study. This type of sampling is very deliberate, and participants are selected because of their ability to validate and clarify (or refute) the relationships of categories in the emerging theory (Strauss and Corbin 1998).

Through this sampling process, researchers identify key participants to provide information related to the ongoing phase of theory development. Once the theory is developed, it can provide a useful format for hypothesis development and testing using quantitative techniques.

Research findings from Reb's study suggest implications for practice. For example, women expressed that communication and support from health care providers was an important source of support. Negative communication experiences increased feelings of isolation. Participants expressed a need for education regarding available support resources. Significant milestones such as therapy completion and fears of recurrence generated distress. Researchers suggested that interventions by advanced practice nurses could potentially alleviate distress. Finally, the study points to further research on interventions to diminish distress (Reb 2007).

Historical Research

Historical research examines accounts of past events to search for truth (Speziale and Carpenter 2007). Nursing researchers conduct historical studies to facilitate understanding of the nursing discipline by giving us insight into our growth as a profession and a better appreciation about decisions that influence practice. Speziale and Carpenter suggest that knowledge about history provides a critical way of knowing. One difference between historical research and the other qualitative methodologies previously discussed is that historical research is built on positivist research traditions such as those discussed in Chapter 4 (Speziale and Carpenter 2007).

Even prior to the emergence of professional nursing, nurses made significant contributions to health care efforts. Context surrounding health care and nursing roles influences the profession's history and is critical to understanding critical events and their impact. Biographical historical research studies aspects of a person's life and contributions such as the impact of Florence Nightingale on nursing education. Social histories explore events and beliefs that surround a time period such as power structures and social status surrounding the development of visiting nurses. Intellectual histories explore the thinking regarding an event such as the development of professional nursing.

While historians do not necessarily follow a set methodology, key steps guide the research process (Lusk 1997; Sweeney 2005). Steps include identifying researchable phenomenon, forming research questions, developing a study title, conducting a literature review, and analysis (Speziale and Carpenter 2007). Historical studies use existing data sources (Lusk 1997) which might include narrative materials and artifacts. Primary sources are documents created by people who participated in the event of interest such as diaries, letters, notes, and meeting minutes. Secondary sources of data are writings and artifacts that others who did not directly participate in the event prepared, such as newspaper accounts, textbooks, and opinions (Lusk 1997; Speziale and Carpenter 2007). When the event is more recent, it is possible to interview individuals who lived the time and event. This type of interview is called an oral history. Validity and reliability of information sources is a significant concern. External criticism is used to determine the authenticity of documents by examining age, type of paper used, and handwriting verification. Internal criticism is the process in which the investigator assesses the reliability of the information (Sweeney 2005). Analysis occurs throughout data collection. Historical studies are more than simply recording information about an event. Histories involve interpretation of the evidence about the event and drawing conclusions about how this information is applicable in current times. Note the history summary in Box 7-12. Not only does it account for the context of the historical influenza pandemic in 1918, it also provides suggestions for management of current day epidemics.

Consider This . . .

If you saw a reproduction of an original document on the Library of Congress site, would you be more inclined to find it trustworthy than if you saw it on Wikipedia? Why or why not?

Case Study Research

Case study research is a qualitative method used to understand how an issue or problem works (Creswell 2007). These problems are called cases, and case studies represent a bounded or limited entity that is explored to increase insight into the issue. Case studies may be instrumental when investigators focus on a specific issue or concern represented by one case. For example, tubing misconnections are a common patient error in nursing that causes harmful outcomes. Studying a particular case may uncover flaws in the system or in nursing actions that permit this error to occur. Collective case studies use several

> ### BOX 7-12   Sample Summary of an Historical Study
>
> Keeling, A. 2010. Alert to the necessities of the emergency: U.S. nursing during the 1918 influenza pandemic. *Public Health Reports, 125*(Supplement 3): 105–112.
>
> In the fall of 1918, the United States found itself in a World War, living in segregated societies, and in the grips of an influenza epidemic. Each of these factors strained the availability of trained nurses, leaving those unfortunate enough to catch influenza without the care and services needed.
>
> Complexities of the situation included the deployment of 9,000 nurses overseas. Use of nurse's aids met resistance from nursing, which had only recently begun to claim professional status obtained through registration and licensure. Military and civilian forces underutilized African-American nurses by limiting or preventing enrollments into nursing programs and requiring nurses recruited for the military nursing corps to have graduated from hospital schools with 50 or more beds. These requirements prevented black nurses educated at smaller hospitals from entering the military.
>
> However, nursing in some respects was prepared to combat the epidemic. Excellent nursing leadership, established programs for public health nurses, and planning for at home emergencies/disasters all played a role in combating influenza. These pieces of infrastructure along with emergency planning enabled nurses to effectively meet demands for nursing care. Preparation for contemporary epidemics should rely on a strong public health infrastructure as well as nationwide planning that includes representatives from nursing as well as medicine and public health.

cases to explore the issue. Researchers attempt to extrapolate from one case information that might be applicable to similar cases or situations. Data collection relies on multiple resources, including document examination, interviews, formal and informal conversations, focus groups, journal excerpts, and phone conversations (Patton 2002). Box 7-13 provides an example of a case study about transformational leadership. A specific case (Florence Wald) and context were used to examine the issue of care for the dying in the post-World War II era. Studying this case provided insight into the problems of terminal care and the evolution of palliative care in the United States. Notice the recommendations for contemporary nurse leaders and the model of transformational leadership.

> ### BOX 7-13   Sample Summary of a Case Study
>
> Adams, C. 2010. Dying with dignity in America: The transformational leadership of Florence Wald. *Journal of Professional Nursing, 26*(2): 125–132.
>
> Following World War II, caring for the dying represented a significant problem that propelled the movement toward the hospice model of care. Florence Wald became a significant force in transforming care through organizing community leaders, clergy, and health care providers. Ultimately, Wald opened the first U.S. hospice in 1971.
>
> To gather information about the case, the researcher used interviews to collect accounts about the historical, psychological, and socio-cultural context in which the evolution of palliative care occurred. Interviews included talking with Florence Wald and six other hospice founders and colleagues. The researcher examined correspondence from archives and a prior interview of Florence Wald.

Wald exhibited a transformational leadership style that examined readiness for change and worked to provide physical, financial, and community support to promote success of a hospice. She built consensus through collaboration with others and asking hard questions about raising the standard of care for the dying.

Contemporary nurse leaders who wish to bring about meaningful change should work to build consensus, bringing about shared values among a wide group of stakeholders. This process creates broad ownership of proposed change and provides a base that will support and maintain successful outcomes.

SUMMARY

In this chapter we explored the five phases of research as they apply to qualitative research and looked at five types of qualitative studies. Key points discussed in this chapter include the following:

- Qualitative research utilizes an inductive process of discovery, moving from specific cases to broader descriptions of phenomenon. The purpose of using qualitative techniques to study problems is to provide a depth of information not feasible in quantitative research. *(Objective 1)*

- Five phases of qualitative research systematically guide the process. Each phase requires researcher decisions that guide the study. The phases represent a cycle that continues the inquiry process, as Figure 7-1 shows. Researchers must conceptualize the problem, design the study, implement the design, analyze the data, and use the results. *(Objective 2)*

- Once the problem is formulated, reviewing the literature is essential to uncover what is known. This process assists in framing the research question. In qualitative research, researchers may conduct an additional literature review at the completion of the analysis process to further examine unanticipated findings.

- Philosophical underpinnings guide selection of research processes, including phenomenology, ethnography, and grounded theory. One of the beliefs of descriptive phenomenology is that the experiences of human beings have a common essence that can be discovered through examination and described. **Hermeneutic** phenomenology, through examination of texts, dialogues, and actions, focuses on describing how the meanings individuals attribute to elements of their world influence their choices. **Symbolic interactionism** provides the theoretical underpinnings for grounded theory and some aspects of ethnography. It focuses on the meanings of symbols, including physical objects, other humans, language, institutions, ideals, or situations, and how those influence decisions about interactions. **Post-modern existential theory** guides some ethnographic research and focuses on understanding the everyday world of human existence.

- Participants are recruited from the field of study. **Purposeful sampling** is used to select research participants who possess first-hand knowledge about the area of study.

- **Rigor** in qualitative research is maintained through ensuring the **trustworthiness** of information. **Credibility** refers to the truthfulness or believability of the findings. **Transferability** reflects the ability to generalize to groups beyond the

study sample. **Dependability** examines how stable or constant qualitative data remain over time. **Confirmability** captures a sense of objectivity in the research.
(Objective 3)

• Special ethical considerations in qualitative research include maintenance of confidentiality, participant–researcher relationships, and sensitivity of some study areas.
(Objective 4)

• In order to successfully conduct qualitative studies, researchers must gain access to
the field by securing permission from institutions, IRBs, and sometimes, informal
gatekeepers.

> • Researchers use multiple methods for data collection. Most commonly used are
> **semi-structured interviewing** and its close cousin **focus group** interviews, par-
> ticipant and nonparticipant observation, and examination of artifacts. Data are
> collected until **saturation** occurs.
> • **Field notes** about events are often kept during the process of data collection.
> Writing **memos** helps researchers track analytic decisions.
> • Examination of written materials and collection of artifacts may supplement
> data collection. *(Objective 5)*

• Analysis of qualitative data is a systematic process that may be completed manually or with computer assistance. Through analysis, researchers identify commonalities and differences in participant accounts about the phenomenon.

> • **Constant comparison** is an analytic strategy that helps researchers systemati-
> cally compare interview data.
> • Once analysis is completed, it is important to present and publish the findings.
> *(Objective 6)*

• There are three major types of qualitative research including (a) **phenomenology**,
(b) **ethnography**, and (c) **grounded theory**. Two additional types of research using narrative data are **historical research** and **case study research**. Each of these
methods has a unique purpose that is directed toward the topic the investigator is
studying.

> • The aim of phenomenology is description.
> • Ethnography provides a description of a culture or group.
> • Grounded theory uses an inductive process to produce a theory.
> • Historical research uses narrative information of past events to better understand
> the present. Historical studies describe events and context as well as providing
> interpretations and deriving implications for contemporary times.
> • Case study research represents a method for investigating a specific issue or
> problem illustrated through study of a case or cases. *(Objective 7)*

Review the questions below, visit the web site, and work the web exercises designed for
this chapter.

STUDENT ACTIVITIES

Now it is time for you to see whether you can apply what you have learned.

1. Hospital stays for women following a mastectomy (breast removal) are very
short. Following mastectomy, women routinely go home with dressings in place
and drains or tubes placed in their surgical incision.

a. As a nurse, what would you want to know about how these women manage their care at home? Make a list of your questions.

b. Would qualitative exploration help to answer the questions on your list?

c. How might this information be useful to nurses?

2. Go to your library resource and use the *CINAHL* (Cumulative Index for Nursing and Allied Health Literature) database. Download two or more of the following qualitative research articles:

Phenomenology: Rodgers, C., A. Young, M. Hockenberry, B. Binder, and L. Symes. 2010. The meaning of adolescents' eating experiences during bone marrow transplant recovery. *Journal of Pediatric Oncology Nursing, 27*(2): 65–72.

Espinosa, L., A. Young, T. Walsh, L. Symes, and B. Binder. 2010. ICU nurse's experiences in providing terminal care. *Critical Care Nursing Quarterly, 33*(3): 273–281.

Ethnography: Stafford, T., M. Myers, A. Young, J. Foster, and J. Huber. 2008. Working in an eICU unit: Life in the Box. *Critical Care Nursing Clinics of North America, 20*(4): 441–450.

Grounded Theory: Greco, K., L. Nail, J. Kendall, J. Cartwright, and D. Messecar. 2010. Mammography decision making in older women with a breast cancer family history. *Journal of Nursing Scholarship, 42*(3): 348–356.

a. Compare the purpose and research methods of the articles.

b. How were data collected?

c. How were data analyzed?

d. Review the findings. Think of at least one or two ways the findings might be relevant to practice.

Pearson Nursing Student Resources

Find additional review materials at

www.nursing.pearsonhighered.com

Prepare for success with additional NCLEX®-style practice questions, interactive assignments and activities, web links, animations and videos, and more!

REFERENCES

Adams, C. 2010. Dying with dignity in America: The transformational leadership of Florence Wald. *Journal of Professional Nursing, 26*(2): 125–132.

Amerson, R. 2010. Facebook: A tool for nursing education research. *Journal of Nursing Education, 50*(7): 414–416.

Beck, C. and S. Watson. 2008. Impact of birth trauma on breast-feeding: A tale of two pathways. *Nursing Research, 57*(4): 228–236.

Benner, P. 1994. The tradition and skill of interpretive phenomenology in studying health, illness, and caring practices. In P. Benner (Ed.), *Interpretive phenom-*

enology: Embodiment, caring and ethics in health and illness (pp. 99–128). Thousand Oaks, CA: Sage.

Birks, M., Y. Chapman, and K. Francis. 2008. Memoing in qualitative research: Probing data and processes. *Journal of Research in Nursing, 13*(1): 68–75.

Blumer, H. 1969. *Symbolic interactionism: Perspectives and method.* Berkley, CA: University of California Press.

Creswell, J.W. 2007. *Qualitative inquiry and research design: Choosing among five approaches* (2nd ed.). Thousand Oaks, CA: Sage.

Eide, P. and D. Kahn. 2008. Ethical issues in the qualitative researcher-participant relationship. *Nursing Ethics, 15*(2): 199–207.

Garcia, C. and E. Saewyc. 2007. Perceptions of mental health among recently immigrated Mexican adolescents. *Issues in Mental Health Nursing, 28*: 37–54.

Gaudine, A., S. LeFort, M. Lamb, and L. Thorne. 2011. Clinical ethical conflicts of nurses and physicians. *Nursing Ethics, 18*(1): 9–19.

Giorgi, A. 1985. *Phenomenology and psychological research.* Pittsburgh, PA: Duquesne University Press.

Glaser, B. and A. Strauss. 1967. *The discovery of grounded theory: Strategies for qualitative research.* New York, NY: Aldine de Gruyter.

Heidegger, M. 1962. *Being and time* (J. Macquarrie and E. Robinson, trans.). New York, NY: Harper & Row.

Heilferty, C. 2011. Ethical considerations in the study of online illness narratives: a qualitative review. *Journal of Advanced Nursing, 67*(5): 945–953.

Hew, K. and W. Cheung. 2008. Attracting student participation in asynchronous online discussions: A case study of peer facilitation. *Computers and Education, 51*(3): 1111–1124.

Hood, L.E., J.K. Olson, and M. Allen. 2007. Learning to care for spiritual needs: Connecting spiritually. Qualitative Health Research, 17(9): 1198–1206.

Hughes, A., M. Gudmundsdottir, and B. Davies. 2007. Everyday struggling to survive: Experiences of the urban poor living with advanced cancer. *Oncology Nursing Forum, 34*(6): 1113–1118.

Husserl, E. 1962. *Ideas: General introduction to pure phenomenology.* (WR Gibson, trans.). New York, NY: Collier Macmillan (originally published in 1932).

Keeling, A. 2010. Alert to the necessities of the emergency: U.S. nursing during the 1918 influenza pandemic. *Public Health Reports, 125*(Supplement 3): 105–112.

Kennedy, E. 2008. Implementing ethically-sound research on online health related support groups. *The Internet Journal of Allied Health Sciences and Practice, 6*(4): 1–8.

Kotarba, J.A. and D. Hurt. 1995. An ethnography of an AIDS hospice: Towards a theory of organizational pastiche. *Symbolic Interaction, 18*(4): 413–438.

Kvale, S. and S. Brinkmann. 2009. *InterViews: Learning the craft of qualitative research interviewing* (2nd ed.). Los Angeles, CA: Sage.

Langford, R. 2001. *Navigating the maze of nursing research.* St. Louis, MO: Mosby.

Lincoln, Y. and E. Guba. (1985). *Naturalistic inquiry.* Newbury Park, CA: Sage.

Lofland, J., D. Snow, L. Anderson, and L. Lofland. 2006. *Analyzing social settings: A guide to qualitative observation and analysis* (4th ed.). Belmont, CA: Wadsworth.

Lopez, K., and D. Willis. 2004. Descriptive versus interpretive phenomenology: Their contributions to nursing knowledge. *Qualitative Health Research, 14*(5): 726–735.

Lusk, B. 1997. Historical methodology for nursing research. *Image: Journal of Nursing Scholarship, 29*(4): 355–360.

Manning, P. 1973. Existential sociology. *Sociological Quarterly, 14*: 200–225.

McGahey-Oakland, P., H. Lieder, A. Young, and L. Jefferson. 2007. Family experiences during resuscitation at a children's hospital emergency department. *Journal of Pediatric Health Care, 21*(4): 217–225.

Patton, M.Q. 2002. *Qualitative research and evaluation methods* (3rd ed.). Thousand Oaks, CA: Sage.

Reb, A. 2007. Transforming the death sentence: Elements of hope in women with advanced ovarian cancer. *Oncology Nursing Forum, 34*(6): E70–E81.

Rodgers, C., A. Young, M. Hockenberry, B. Binder, and L. Symes. 2010. The meaning of adolescents' eating experiences during bone marrow transplant recovery. *Journal of Pediatric Oncology Nursing, 27*(2): 65–72.

Snyder, B. 2006. The lived experience of women diagnosed with polycystic ovary syndrome. *Journal of Obstetric, Gynecology, and Neonatal Nursing, 35*(3): 385–392.

Speziale, H. and D. Carpenter. 2007. *Qualitative research in nursing: Advancing the humanistic imperative* (4th ed.). Philadelphia, PA: Lippincott Williams & Wilkins.

Spradley, J. 1979. *The ethnographic interview.* New York, NY: Holt, Rinehart, and Winston.

Stafford, T., M. Myers, A. Young, J. Foster, and J. Huber. 2008. Working in an eICU unit: Life in the Box. *Critical Care Nursing Clinics of North America, 20*(4): 441–450.

Strauss, A. and J. Corbin. 1998. *Basics of qualitative research: Techniques and procedures for developing grounded theory* (2nd ed.). Thousand Oaks, CA: Sage.

Sweeney, J. 2005. Historical research: Examining documentary resources. *Nurse Researcher, 12*(3): 61–73.

Symes, L. 2000. Arriving at readiness to recover emotionally after sexual assault. *Archives of Psychiatric Nursing, 14*(1): 30–30.

Townsend, A., S. Cox, and L. Li. 2010. Qualitative research ethics: Enhancing evidence-based practice in physical therapy. *Physical Therapy, 90*(4): 615–628.

How Do I Use What I Know?

. . . effectively reading research articles, identifying evidence,

applying research evidence to clinical problems

B est practices demand that we use the most current and relevant information available. To use such information you need to know how to read and evaluate it. This section is designed to let you develop and practice your skills as a research consumer. It will help you learn to apply research findings to your own clinical practice. In these chapters you will examine the standard research article layout and be introduced to a reading strategy that will allow you to survey, examine, and evaluate such research articles. You will learn about the concept of evidence based practice (EBP) and its utility in addressing clinical problems. You will investigate how to design and implement an evidence-based project using the research literature. Finally you will put the whole picture together as you see an EBP unfold before your eyes.

Using Critical Reading Skills to Evaluate Research

CHAPTER OBJECTIVES

1. Describe standard elements of journal formats used to present research studies.
2. Discuss the functions of standard elements contained in an article.
3. Describe a strategy designed to increase effective reading of research studies.
4. Use the SEE (Survey, Examine, and Evaluate) strategy to survey an article to discern its aims and structure.
5. Apply the SEE strategy to examine qualitative and quantitative research studies.
6. Use the SEE process to assist in determining the usefulness of research studies in clinical settings.

KEY TERMS

Abstract (p. 160)

Critical reading (p. 164)

Discussion (p. 164)

Evaluate (p. 181)

Examine (p. 168)

Introduction (p. 161)

Methods (p. 162)

References (p. 164)

Research critique (p. 181)

Results (p. 163)

SEE method (p. 164)

Survey (p. 165)

ABSTRACT

*The journal articles through which most researchers disseminate their results generally include common elements in a format that includes a title and abstract, introduction, methods, results, discussion, and references. These sections reflect the steps of the research process. Using a systematic reading strategy improves understanding and application of research findings. The SEE reading strategy described in this chapter consists of three phases: The **survey** phase uncovers the general purpose of the study. The **examine** phase focuses on identifying core ideas and key elements of the research process. The **evaluate** phase determines the usefulness of the material and envisions the use of study results in practice.*

Reading and understanding research are both critical steps in locating and using evidence to guide nursing practice. While reading research may seem intimidating at first, this chapter will help to break the process down into smaller pieces to make it more approachable. We divide the chapter into two major areas. First, we describe a typical format for published research findings. Second, we present a strategy for critically reading, understanding, and applying the findings from published quantitative and qualitative research articles.

Components of Research Articles

Research studies are most widely disseminated through professional journals. We have already identified several research and clinical journals focusing on the presentation of nursing research studies. As you have undoubtedly noticed when previewing some of these resources, the presentation format for research articles is relatively similar regardless of the journal. Although this format evolved from a strong quantitative research tradition, qualitative research studies follow it as well. A research article is generally comprised of six major sections:

- Title and Abstract
- Introduction or Background
- Methodology
- Results or Findings
- Discussion or Conclusions
- References

Consider This . . .

Think about a research article you have seen. What did you notice about the structure of the article? In what ways did the article headings give you clues about what you might find?

Though the titles may vary somewhat, the major sections are usually recognizable across journals. Qualitative articles generally follow this format to provide consistency in journal presentation, yet as qualitative research finds broader acceptance in nursing, we are beginning to see presentations that are more suited to the nature of the qualitative process. This is particularly evident in journals that specialize in the publication of qualitative research studies. Table 8-1 summarizes the location of the various parts of the research process in this format structure.

Let us examine each of these six sections more closely to see what to expect when reading a research article.

Title and Abstract

The study title, set off in boldfaced large print, is designed to attract attention. The title should capture the essence of the study. It typically states the variables or phenomena of interest and the study population. The first encounter with the study title usually occurs when conducting a search of available literature on a subject of interest. Readers of research use the title to decide whether a study is relevant or unrelated to the focus of their search. The title section also lists the names and credentials of the researchers who conducted the study. This information can help readers to judge the researchers' qualifications. For example, are the investigators nurses or a part of a multidisciplinary team? Do the authors' educational and clinical credentials indicate that they have potentially relevant academic and clinical knowledge to conduct the study?

Abstracts typically fall just below the title and sometimes are set off in italicized print. The **abstract** provides a concise summary of the study, giving an overview of the article and a preview of the research findings. An abstract briefly describes the study purpose, research design, methodology, and findings in 100–300 words. The format of the abstract may vary from publication to publication. Some journals call for a very concise paragraph not to exceed 150 words. Other journals employ a more comprehensive approach, and the abstract may offer a summary of each of the major study sections (such as the study objectives, methods, results, and conclusions). This more comprehensive form may run up to 300 words.

Abstracts further assist in making decisions about the relevance of a given article during a library search, as we discussed in Chapter 2. An abstract clearly related to the

▶ **Table 8-1   Placement of Research Process Components in Journal Format**

Article Sections	Research Process
Title and Abstract	
Introduction or Background	Problem statement/purpose
	Literature review
	Theoretical framework
	Hypotheses/research questions
	Objectives/study aims
Methods	Research design
	Sample and setting
	Data collection procedures
	Data analysis procedures
Results or Findings	Description of sample
	Presentation of results
Discussion or Conclusions	Interpretation of results
	Recommendations for research
	Implications for nursing
References	

subject under consideration should lead you to retrieve a copy of the full article. Some journals also list key terms immediately under the abstract. These terms conform to subject headings in databases such as *CINAHL* or MEDLINE. Using these key terms may help you to refine your search parameters.

Introduction or Background

The **introduction** is the first section in the body of the article, although it often contains no section head. It presents the background for the study and acquaints readers with the research problem and its context. It explains why it is important to study the problem. Descriptions of several key elements of the research process reside in this section, including the research problem, research questions or hypotheses, a review of literature, and the theoretical framework. These elements may appear under titled subheads or may be interwoven into the section as a whole.

The introduction often begins with a statement about the need for the research, followed by a brief presentation of current literature. Because of space constraints, the literature review cannot mention every available resource. Rather, it cites only the most critical and current studies. Sometimes the discussion section contains additional literature review. The introduction section may also present a guiding theoretical framework. However, many published research articles do not explicitly state their underlying theory.

The research problem statement is usually located at the end of the introductory section. The research problem can be identified by terms such as *study purpose, objectives, aims,* or *focus*. The problem may then be broken down into smaller segments identified as research questions or hypotheses. The introduction to a study should give readers a good feel for what is being studied and why such a study is important.

Methodology

The **methods** section describes how researchers carried out the study. This section usually identifies the research design and describes the subjects, sampling techniques, setting, data collection process, and data analysis procedures. Research journals generally place a greater emphasis on this section than do clinical journals. Journals may use subheadings in this section that assist readers to more easily locate information.

RESEARCH DESIGN. A description of the research design and the rationale for its selection are usually located at the beginning of the methods section. With experimental studies, the design description contains greater detail and specificity (review Chapter 6 regarding quantitative research designs). Readers need to know how the research situation was controlled and what variables were manipulated. This information helps readers make judgments about possible threats to the internal validity of the study. Design descriptions in quantitative non-experimental studies may be much briefer simply because fewer elements are controlled. Qualitative studies may present a brief statement about the type of study and the philosophical underpinnings in this section. These studies frequently elaborate on the design tradition (Chapter 7 describes qualitative designs). For example, a grounded theory study might describe the specific characteristics of the grounded theory approach.

SAMPLE AND SETTING. The methods section often contains information about study participants. Subtitles used in this section may include sample, subjects, participants, or setting. Here you will find a discussion of the sample, sample size, sampling techniques, and the setting for the study. Quantitative studies often list inclusion and/or exclusion criteria used in sample selection. There may also be a discussion of response rates and attrition of subjects. Qualitative studies will address the selection of participants using specific, purposive selection methods. A more detailed description of the setting may also appear in qualitative studies. Information about the sample and sampling plan allows readers to make judgments about appropriate application of the study results. Sometimes this section makes reference to protection of human subjects; however, this information is sometimes omitted due to space constraints in the journal. Although, in some instances, articles may have an explicit heading identifying ethical considerations.

DATA COLLECTION. The next methods subsection describes how the researchers collected their data. Sometimes this section is broken into subsections labeled as data collection, instruments, or variables/measures. Quantitative studies list and briefly describe the instruments used to measure study variables and report any pertinent reliability and validity levels for those instruments. This section sometimes offers a description of the data collectors and their expertise or training. Experimental studies will provide a description of the intervention administered to the treatment group. Qualitative studies may describe interview or observational techniques and report on the use of data collection measures such as audio-taping interviews and recording field notes or keeping diaries. A discussion of the trustworthiness or credibility of the data should report on the use of audit trails, member checks, peer debriefings, or triangulation (Chapter 7 discusses these items in greater detail).

DATA ANALYSIS. Finally, the methods section should contain a description of the data analysis procedures. In quantitative studies, this description is usually brief, typically identifying the statistical procedures used and the set level of significance. In studies that employ commonly used statistical procedures, this information is often integrated in the results section rather than reported in the methods section. In qualitative studies, the data analysis subsection receives major attention and generally contains a detailed description of the analysis process. This description allows readers to see how data were organized, examined, and synthesized to produce meaningful themes or patterns.

Results or Findings

The results or findings section forms the heart of the article. The **results** section reports the answers to research questions or study aims. Often, the terms results and findings are used interchangeably. The findings section typically provides readers with a description of study participants and presents the key research findings. Possible subheadings include sample characteristics and study results/findings. Qualitative studies frequently organize the findings section by using subheadings to identify themes found during analysis.

Consider This . . .

If you are having a hard time understanding the results or findings section, what could you do? Whom do you know with enough knowledge to help you?

SAMPLE CHARACTERISTICS. The description of the study participants usually consid-ers such basic characteristics as gender, age, and race, as well as a description of other pertinent characteristics relevant to the study. Quantitative studies often summarize and present this information in tabular form, detailing frequencies and percentages of various variable categories. Reporting measures of central tendency and measures of dispersion adds detail to the sample description, as we saw in Chapter 6. Such descriptions help readers form a more complete picture about the study participants and whether they are similar to individuals seen in their own practice arena.

Qualitative studies should also describe the characteristics of the participants, although they may do so in a narrative manner. Qualitative sample descriptions should offer a clear picture of the study participants. For example, qualitative studies may share the number of participants, their ethnicity, and ages using numbers, as the examples in Chapter 7 show. However, these studies may be less concerned with details such as measures of central tendency and dispersion.

STUDY RESULTS/FINDINGS. The focus of the results section centers on answering the re-search questions or hypotheses. This section is where readers find out the bottom line. In quantitative studies, the results section is fairly short. Data presentation occurs in succinct statistical formats with little discussion. You will see the identification of the statistical test(s) employed, the values of the calculated statistic, and its probability reported. Tables or graphs display much of the statistical information. A brief narrative may translate these statistical results into words.

In experimental studies, researchers want to find out whether the tested intervention was effective. In other words, was the outcome for the treatment group different from the control group? Non-experimental studies want to answer the research questions: How did the variables reveal themselves in the study sample? Were the variables related to or different from one another? If the results section contains complex and difficult-to-understand statistical results, do not give up in your search for the answer to the questions raised by the study. Keep reading and you will find a translation of the statistical results in narrative form.

In qualitative studies the findings section is generally longer. Results appear in narrative form and researchers often use the section to describe the themes, processes, or structures that emerged from the analysis. For example, phenomenological studies may present thematic categories that describe the phenomenon studied. Grounded theory studies use this section to present the theory that has emerged from the data analysis. Novice readers often find the results of qualitative studies much easier to read and understand because they use narrative analysis rather than statistical techniques.

Discussion or Conclusions

Discussion is the process whereby researchers talk about the study findings and tie study outcomes to prior research. Sometime the Discussion section is labeled Conclusions, but regardless of the title, this section focuses on interpreting and making sense of the results. In quantitative studies, the section typically begins with a summary of the study findings. Researchers tie the findings to the research problem described in the introduction. Following a discussion of the meaning of the results, researchers compare findings to the existing body of literature and back to the theoretical framework supporting the study. Researchers should explain unexpected findings (e.g., the hypotheses were not supported) and share study limitations. Implications for nursing practice and recommendations for further research also appear here.

The discussion section in qualitative studies must also address the study problem and discuss findings in light of existing literature. Because transferability is a limiting factor of qualitative research, researchers may limit the implications for nursing practice.

References

Journal articles conclude with a listing of references. The **reference** section lists journal articles, books, and other sources cited in the text of the article. Reference sections are very valuable tool to readers who are interested in further information on a given area of study. It provides a starting point for a preliminary review of the literature on that topic (see Chapter 2). Pay attention to the publications dates of references. They can help you to decide if references are out of date. Keep in mind, though, that some older references are classics that provide foundational work in the field.

Consider This . . .

As a reader, how might you determine if an article is out of date or if it is a classic?

Survey, Examine, and Evaluate

The primary reason for reading research articles is to determine whether the findings will help your professional practice. Using a systematic strategy makes the process of reading articles more fruitful. This process is called **critical reading**. The strategy that we are going to use is the **SEE method** (for Survey, Examine, and Evaluate). Figure 8-1 presents an overview of the strategy.

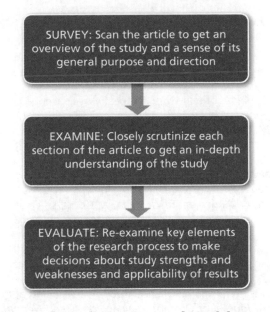

■ **FIGURE 8-1** Steps of Reading a Research Article
Use the SEE strategy to critically read a research article.

Survey

The critical reader's first step is to **survey** the article, scanning it for general understanding. Pay particular attention to the title, abstract, and references. Look at the title first, noting the study variables or phenomena it identifies. Can you determine the study type? Check the list of authors and author qualifications.

CHECK THE TITLE. Let us examine the information gleaned from a title. Box 8-1 lists several recently published research studies from a variety of research and clinical journals. There are five qualitative studies and five quantitative studies. Can you tell which is which based on the titles (see the answer key on page 192)? Identification for some is easy. For example, consider the title *Living alone with dementia: An interpretive phenomenological study with older women*. Clearly, this is a qualitative phenomenological study. Another title that clearly indicates the study type is *Effects of a physical activity intervention for women*. We know just by glancing that this is a quantitative experimental study because the title tells us that the study tested an intervention (treatment). Less clear is the title *Voices of midwives: A tapestry of challenges and blessings*. It sounds as if the study is qualitative, but you will need to assess the abstract to know for certain. What about *An exercise program to improve fall-related outcomes in elderly nursing home residents* or *Supplementing relaxation and music for pain after surgery*? These titles imply that a treatment was tested, but once again you will need to skim the abstract to confirm whether these two studies are in fact experimental in design.

Now let's use the titles to gather information about the focus of the study. In the phenomenological study *Living alone with dementia: An interpretive phenomenological study with older women*, you can tell from the title that the researchers' sample was older women with mild to moderate Alzheimer's disease or dementia who lived alone. The study focused on the meaning of the phenomenon of living at home alone with this mental impairment. In the quantitative study *An exercise program to improve fall-related*

> ## BOX 8-1   Research Article Titles
>
> deWitt, L., J. Ploeg, and M. Black. 2010. Living alone with dementia: An interpretive phenomenological study with older women. *Journal of Advanced Nursing, 66*(8): 1698–1707.
>
> Doherty, M.E. 2010. Voices of midwives: A tapestry of challenges and blessings. *MCN: The American Journal of Maternal Child Nursing, 35*(2): 96–101.
>
> El-Masri, M.M., S.M. Fox-Wasylyshyn, and T.A. Hammad. 2005. Predicting nosocomial bloodstream infections using surrogate markers of injury severity. *Nursing Research, 54*(4): 273–279.
>
> Garcia, C. and E. Saewyc. 2007. Perceptions of mental health among recently immigrated Mexican adolescents. *Issues in Mental Health Nursing, 28:* 37–54.
>
> Good, M., J. Gilbert, G. Anderson, S. Wotman, X. Cong, D. Lane, and S. Ahn. 2010. Supplementing relaxation and music for pain after surgery. *Nursing Research, 59*(4): 259–269.
>
> Greco, K., L. Nail, J. Kendall, J. Cartwright, and D. Messecar. 2010. Mammography decision making in older women with a breast cancer family history. *Journal of Nursing Scholarship, 42*(3): 348–356.
>
> MacKinnon, K., M. McIntyre, and M. Quance. 2005. The meaning of the nurse's presence during childbirth. *Journal of Obstetric, Gynecologic, and Neonatal Nursing, 34*(3): 28–36.
>
> Newhouse, R.P., M. Johantgen, P.J. Pronovost, and E. Johnson. 2005. Perioperative nurses and patient outcomes-mortality, complications, and length of stay. *AORN Journal, 81*(3): 508–509, 513–516, 518, 520–522, 525–528.
>
> Peterson, J.A., B.C. Yates, J.R. Atwood, and M. Hertzog. 2005. Effects of a physical activity intervention for women. *Western Journal of Nursing Research, 27*(1): 93–110.
>
> Schoenfelder, D.P. and L.M. Rubenstein. 2004. An exercise program to improve fall-related outcomes in elderly nursing home residents. *Applied Nursing Research, 17*(1): 21–31.

outcomes in elderly nursing home residents, the sample is nursing home residents and the variables under study are exercise and falls. The study title *Effects of a physical activity intervention for women* is more general. The sample is women and physical activity is one variable under study, but we do not really know at this point what type of women or what specific effects of exercise are being studied. What did you learn about the sample and variables or phenomena in the other articles in Box 8-1?

SCAN THE ABSTRACT. After checking the title, perusing the abstract can help you to determine or confirm the study type, identify the study objective(s), see the methodology employed, and determine the study's bottom line. Let's look at abstracts from two of the cited studies. Box 8-2 shows the abstracts for two of the articles listed in Box 8-1: a quantitative study (Schoenfelder and Rubenstein 2004) and a qualitative study (Mackinnon, McIntyre, and Quance 2005). These samples illustrate two types of abstracts that you are likely to encounter when reading research: a single paragraph summary and a more structured synopsis that uses specific headings to highlight key sections.

   In the study investigating an exercise program to improve fall-related outcomes in elderly nursing home residents, the Schoenfelder and Rubenstein abstract clearly informs us that the study is experimental (*exercise group vs. control group*). It identifies

BOX 8-2 Sample of Quantitative and Qualitative Abstracts

Quantitative Abstract

An exercise program to improve fall-related outcomes in elderly nursing home residents.

"This study tested a 3-month ankle-strengthening and walking program designed to improve or maintain the fall-related outcomes of balance, ankle strength, walking speed, risk of falling, fear of falling, and confidence to perform daily activities without falling (falls efficacy) in elderly nursing home residents. Nursing home residents ($N = 81$) between the ages of 64 and 100 years participated in the study. Two of the fall-related outcomes, balance and fear of falling, were maintained or improved for the exercise group in comparison to the control group" (p. 21).

Schoenfelder, D.P. and L.M. Rubenstein. 2004. An exercise program to improve fall-related outcomes in elderly nursing home residents. *Applied Nursing Research, 17*(1): 21–31.

Qualitative Abstract

The meaning of the nurse's presence during childbirth.

"Objective: The purpose of this exploratory study was to develop new understandings of what it means to women in labor for a nurse to be present during childbirth.

Design: Hermeneutic inquiry was used to explore the phenomenon of nursing presence during childbirth. The purpose of questioning in hermeneutic phenomenology is to stimulate thoughtful reflection and deeper exploration of the subject's experiences.

Participants/Setting: Six women from an urban center in Canada volunteered to share their experiences of childbirth through conversations with the research team.

Data Analysis: Audio-taped, transcribed interviews were analyzed along with the reflections of the research team.

Results: Women attribute multiple meanings to the care provided by intrapartum nurses. However, what stood out in these women's accounts was that a nurse's presence was the way in which a nurse was "there" for them and was a very important part of their childbirth experience" (p. 28).

MacKinnon, K., M. McIntyre, and M. Quance, 2005. The meaning of the nurse's presence during childbirth. *Journal of Obstetric, Gynecologic, and Neonatal Nursing, 34*(1): 28–36.

---

a treatment (*3-month ankle-strengthening and walking program*) and delineates the anticipated outcomes (*improve or maintain the fall-related outcomes*). It briefly describes the sample (*81 nursing home residents between the ages of 64 and 100*) and reveals the bottom line (*balance and fear of falling were maintained or improved for the exercise group*) (Schoenfelder and Rubenstein 2004, p. 21).

In the qualitative study that researched the meaning of the nurse's presence during childbirth, the MacKinnon team notes in their abstract the use of a phenomenological design (*hermeneutic phenomenology*). The study objective is clearly identified with a specific heading and succinctly states the study purpose (*to develop new understandings of what it means to women in labor for a nurse to be present during childbirth*). Participants/Setting and Data Analysis are also identified as headings and provide a brief identification of the sample (*six women from an urban center in Canada*) and data collection measures (*audio-taped, transcribed interviews*).

The results provide us with a glimpse of the findings (*what stood out in these women's accounts was that a nurse's presence was the way in which a nurse was "there" for them and was a very important part of their childbirth experience*) (MacKinnon et al. 2005, p. 28).

SKIM THE TEXT AND REFERENCES. The next step in the survey process is to skim the major sections of the full text of the article. The purpose here is to glean the study highlights. Don't get bogged down by details, unfamiliar terms, or confusing statistical treatments. Rather, familiarize yourself with the study to get the big picture. The final step of surveying the article is to scan the reference list and to determine whether any of the cited articles might be helpful in your exploration of the topic. You may want to make a note to pull those articles whose titles look promising, as described in Chapter 2.

Examine

The next phase of the SEE process is to **examine** the text of the article section by section to gain a better understanding of the study. This examination is broken down for each major section of the research article.

INTRODUCTION OR BACKGROUND. An article's introduction tells you more about the study problem and its context. To examine this section of an article, follow the process below (Figure 8-2) to gather information regarding the study. Determining who and what

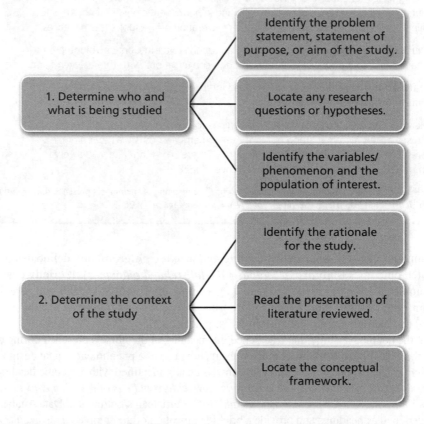

■ FIGURE 8-2 Process for Examining Introduction or Background
You can learn a great deal about an article from its introduction.

BOX 8-3 Excerpts from the Introduction of a Quantitative Article

"Older adults who reside in nursing homes often have multiple health risks, including the risk of falling with the resultant potential for injury. Frail elders who fall are likely to fall repeatedly, further increasing their risk for serious injury. Fractures, injury and immobility may lead to . . . disability or death. The fear of falling . . . inhibit[s] physical activities . . . and compromise[s] quality of life. . . . Results of a pilot study suggested that a walking and ankle-strengthening program could improve fall-related outcomes and prevent or slow physical deterioration in elderly nursing home residents. . . . This follow-up study investigated the effectiveness of an ankle-strengthening and walking program for elderly nursing home residents in improving . . . fall-related outcomes" (p. 21).

"Although elderly nursing home residents are at a great risk for falling and deterioration of physical and functional abilities, this population has not been studied extensively to test the effects of exercise on fall-related outcomes" (p 23).

"The researchers hypothesized that the proportion of elders with consistent or improved fall-related outcomes would be significantly higher for those individuals participating in the ankle-strengthening and walking program than for those elders who did not participate. The fall-related outcomes for this study were balance, ankle strength, walking speed, falls risk, fear of falling, and confidence to perform daily activities without falling (falls efficacy)" (p 23).

(Excerpted from Schoenfelder and Rubenstein 2004)

is being studied helps you better understand the researcher's intent and adds information regarding study variables. Learning more about the contextual elements of the study helps explain why the study is important—specifically what the study contributes to the knowledge base—and places the research in a theoretical perspective.

Let's examine the introductions of the quantitative and qualitative studies we've been reading to find out more detail about what and who the researchers studied. Box 8-3 contains excerpts from the introduction and background section of the Schoenfelder article on falls and Box 8-4 contains excerpts from the MacKinnon article on the nurse's presence during childbirth.

Let's apply the process laid out in Figure 8-2 to the study in Box 8-3. The problem statement appears at the end of the first paragraph: "... *investigated the effectiveness of an ankle-strengthening and walking program for elderly nursing home residents in improving . . . fall-related outcomes.*" The paragraph that begins "the researchers hypothesized" makes it easy to spot the hypothesis: "... *the proportion of elders with consistent or improved fall-related outcomes would be significantly higher for those individuals participating in the ankle-strengthening and walking program than for those elders who did not participate.*" The independent variable is *"ankle-strengthening and walking program"* and the dependent variable is *"fall-related outcomes."* The introduction nicely breaks down the dependent variable into its component parts *("balance, ankle strength, walking speed, falls risk, fear of falling, and confidence to perform daily activities without falling")*. There is a clear statement of the population of interest in the first sentence: *"Older adults who reside in nursing homes . . ."* (Schoenfelder and Rubenstein 2004, pp. 21–23).

The opening paragraph of the introduction also succinctly reveals the rationale and significance of the study, while the third paragraph expands on it when it states

> ## BOX 8-4 Excerpts from the Introduction of a Qualitative Article
>
> "Recent research has called into question the ability of intrapartum nurses to provide labor support during childbirth . . . we are concerned that the results of this randomized controlled trial could be interpreted to mean that fewer registered nurses are needed to care for women in labor. There is a danger that the generalizing effects of these trials can silence the voices of individual women. This qualitative study of women's experiences of nursing presence during childbirth allows other voices to be heard by perinatal nurses and decision makers" (p. 28).
>
> "The overall purpose of this exploratory study was to develop new understandings of what it means for a nurse to be present during childbirth. Exploring what the presence of an intra-partum nurse means to a woman in labor is important because of the significance of birth in women's lives and the documented influence of labor support on birth outcomes . . . Although supportive care during labor has been shown to decrease the likelihood of medication for pain relief, operative delivery, and low 5-minute Apgar scores in the newborn . . . other research indicates that supportive nursing care is not consistently provided for women in labor . . ." (p. 29).
>
> "The primary research question addressed in this study was 'What meanings do women in labor attribute to the intrapartum nurse's presence during their childbirth experience' " (p. 30)?
>
> (Excerpted from Mackinnon, McIntyre, and Quance 2005)

"*this population has not been studied extensively.*" Though not included in the excerpt, the study also had a brief review of literature. No theoretical or conceptual framework is identified, discussed, or implied for this study.

Now, let's examine the introduction to MacKinnon's qualitative article illustrated in Box 8-4, once again applying the process laid out on page 168 in Figure 8-2. The problem appears as a purpose statement, which clearly indicates the researchers' intent: "*The overall purpose of this exploratory study was to develop new understandings of what it means for a nurse to be present during childbirth.*" The introductory section ends by posing a research question "*What meanings do women in labor attribute to the intrapartum nurse's presence during their childbirth experience?*" It is easy to tell that the phenomenon being studied is *meanings attached to nurse presence*. The population of interest is woman experiencing childbirth (MacKinnon et al. 2005, p. 29).

The first two paragraphs of the excerpt give the context for the research, including a statement of rationale and need for the study (". . . *we are concerned that the results of this randomized controlled trial could be interpreted to mean that fewer registered nurses are needed to care for women in labor*"). A literature review is also included in this study that will not be examined here. Because it is a qualitative study, it does not include a theoretical framework.

METHODS. The methods section of a research study includes valuable information about the conduct of the study and the way the researchers collected and analyzed the data. Figure 8-3 details a step-by-step process for examining researchers' methods discussion. The research design provided an overall plan that guided the implementation of the study. Design features share information about any interventions or treatments used in the study. Sample information informs readers about the nature of the sample and the sample selection process while the setting provides information about the study environment.

Descriptions of data collection methods help readers to discern whether researchers used techniques such as self-reports, observations, or physiological instruments and the specific measures used for the study.

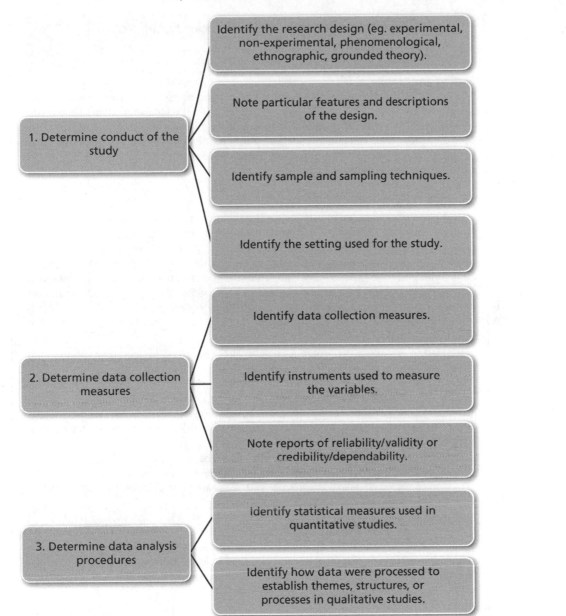

■ FIGURE 8-3 Process for Examining Researchers' Methods Discussions
The Methods section includes valuable information about how researchers conducted the
study and collected and analyzed the data.

Let us continue our examination of our sample articles, turning our attention to the
methods sections for the quantitative (Schoenfelder and Rubenstein 2004) and qualitative
(MacKinnon et al. 2005) studies. Box 8-5 contains excerpts from the methods section of
the quantitative article and Box 8-6 contains excerpts from the qualitative article.

Using the process found in Figure 8-3 to examine the methods section of the quantitative study, we can see that the study used an experimental design even though there

BOX 8-5 Summary Excerpts from Methods Section of Quantitative Article

Setting and Sample

"The study was conducted in 10 private, urban nursing homes in eastern Iowa, ranging in size from 68 to 178 beds" (p. 23). All residents who met the following criteria were invited to participate: at least 65 years old; able to ambulate independently or with an assistive device; no reported unstable physical condition, terminal illness, or history of acting-out behavior; and a score of 20 or more on the Mini-Mental State Examination. Eighty-one subjects completed the study.

Procedure

"Participants were matched in pairs by the Risk Assessment for Falls Scale II scores and then randomly assigned within each pair to the intervention or control group. . . . Subjects assigned to the intervention group participated in a 3-month ankle-strengthening and walking program . . . The 3-month supervised exercising was done three times weekly for about 15 to 20 minutes each time" (pp. 23–24). Subjects in the control group received no exercise intervention but did receive an attention placebo and were visited weekly where 30 minutes was devoted to an activity such as book reading or "friendly visiting."

Instrumentation

Fear of falling was measured by asking subjects "How concerned are you about falling?" Test-retest reliability was acceptable (Kappa = 0.66).

Balance was measured by a stopwatch for up to 10 seconds in three stances: parallel, semi tandem, and tandem. Reliability coefficients ranged from 0.57 to 0.96.

Ankle plantar flexion strength was measured using mechanical force transducer that was calibrated for accuracy by a technical expert from the Instrument Shop where it was manufactured.

Walking speed, the time to walk six meters was measured in seconds with a stopwatch.

Fall-Risk Assessment was measured by the RAFS II, a 13-item tool that provides an indication of the risk of falling. Use in three extended care facilities found the tool to be 90% accurate for predicting falls.

"Falls efficacy was measured by using a modified Falls Efficacy Scale (FES), . . . a 10-item tool designed to assess the degree of perceived self-confidence for avoiding a fall during each of 10 relatively nonhazardous activities of daily living routinely performed by community dwelling elders. Expert validation was accomplished by reaching consensus among therapists, nurses, and physicians concerning the activities to include in the FES" (p. 25). Internal consistency was examined (Cronbach's alpha = 0.9).

Data Analysis

"Data were collected for all variables at baseline, 3 months, and 6 months. Comparisons were made between the intervention and control groups. . . . Tests for group differences used chi square or Fisher's Exact tests for categorical data and either a t test (normal distributions) or Kruskal-Wallace (nonnormal distribution) test for continuous data" (p. 25).

(Excerpted and summarized from Schoenfelder and Rubenstein 2004) is no design specified. The first clue comes at the end of the introduction with the statement of the hypothesis: *"the proportion of elders with consistent or improved fall related outcomes would be significantly higher for those individuals participating in the ankle-strengthening and walking program than for those elders who did not participate."* This tells us that the study used two comparison groups. The statement *"Participants were matched in pairs by the Risk Assessment for Falls Scale II scores and then randomly assigned within each pair to the intervention or control group"* specifies random assignment of subjects to an experimental or control group, the hallmark of an experimental study. Additionally, the intervention for the experimental group versus that received by the control group is specified: *"Subjects assigned to the intervention group participated in a 3-month ankle-strengthening and walking program . . . The 3-month supervised exercising was done three times weekly for about 15 to 20 minutes each time. Subjects in the control group received no exercise intervention but did receive an attention placebo and were visited weekly where 30 minutes was devoted to an activity such as book reading or 'friendly visiting' "* (Schoenfelder and Rubenstein 2004, p. 23).

The section on setting and sample identifies the sampling techniques and inclusion criteria: "All residents who met the following criteria were invited to participate: ..." This section also indicated the number of subjects who completed the study as eighty-one. The setting was described: *"This study was conducted in 10 private, urban nursing homes in eastern Iowa, ranging in size from 68-178 beds"* (Schoenfelder and Rubenstein 2004, p. 23).

As we can see from the Instrumentation section, the researchers used six measures to collect data, including self-report, observation, and physiological measures: (1) Fear of falling: (Self-report); (2) Balance: (Observation); (3) Ankle plantar flexion strength: (Physiological); (4) Walking speed: (Observation); (5) Fall risk assessment: (Observation); and (6) Falls efficacy: (Self-report). See Box 8-5 for more details on each of these instruments. Finally, researchers report the reliability and validity of each of the six measures. Often such reports appear in the form of statistical measures such as a Kappa score or reliability coefficients, or as a description of specific tests run to establish other aspects of reliability and validity. What test for reliability and validity do you see in the Instrumentation section found in Box 8-5 of the Schoenfelder and Rubenstein study?

Readers can find information about frequency of data collection in the Data Analysis section: *"Data were collected for all variables at baseline, 3 months, and 6 months"* (Schoenfelder and Rubenstein 2004, p. 25). The Data Analysis section also identifies the statistical comparisons made between the intervention and control groups. See the Data Analysis section of Box 8-5 for more details on each of these instruments. Note the tests for group differences.

Applying the process in Figure 8-3 for the Methods section to the excerpts from the qualitative study reveals that the investigators clearly identify their study as qualitative: it is *"A hermeneutic phenomenological inquiry. . . ."* The researchers' detailed description of the design in the Method section helps readers who may not be familiar with the hermeneutic approach understand that *". . . this method of study is important for understanding everyday experiences that may be invisible or unseen."* In order to give readers a clear picture of how they used the hermeneutic design, investigators offer a specific explanation of the design application: *"For intrapartum nurses, birth is such a common experience that it is easy to take its meanings for granted. For the woman, giving birth is unique and emotional. These conversations explored the tension between the intrapartum nurse's experiences of birth as a routine occurrence and the woman's desire for a special birth experience. . .*" Note there is no discussion of interventions because the intent of this method is to describe what currently exists rather than measure the effects of a specific treatment (MacKinnon et al. 2005, pp. 30–31).

The Participants/Setting section discusses the mechanism used for sample acquisition. Note how small the sample is when compared to quantitative studies: "*Six women volunteered to participate.*" It describes how sample selection focuses on women who had experienced childbirth in the last 6 months and met the study inclusion criteria. Information about the setting is limited to the location: "*. . . from an urban center in Canada*" (MacKinnon et al. 2005, p. 31).

BOX 8-6 Summary Excerpts from Methods Section of a Qualitative Article

Method/Design
"A hermeneutic phenomenological inquiry involves the generation of meanings through the interpretation of texts. In this research, the primary texts were those generated through conversational, audio-taped interviews with study participants. . . .Drawing on hermeneutic philosophy, part of the intention of this research is to create a clearing or a space around the woman's experience of the nurse's presence so that a conversation about what is going on may occur . . . Specifically, this method of study is important for understanding everyday experiences that may be invisible or unseen. For intrapartum nurses, birth is such a common experience that it is easy to take its meanings for granted. For the woman, giving birth is unique and emotional. These conversations explored the tension between the intrapartum nurse's experiences of birth as a routine occurrence and the woman's desire for a special birth experience . . . After encouraging women to describe their recent childbirth experience, women in this study were asked, "What was it like for you to have a nurse present during your labor and birth" (p. 30)?

Participants/Setting
"A purposive sample was recruited from an urban center in Canada. Participants were volunteers, who wanted to share their stories about nursing presence during their recent, particular birth experiences" . . . and "were selected by virtue of their status as expert witnesses to their experiences during childbirth, were at least 18-years old, were able to speak English fluently, and were interviewed during the first 6 months after childbirth. . . . Six women volunteered to participate" (p. 31).

Data Analysis
"Interviews were conducted by two members of the research team who also reflected on the nonverbal cues that were part of the research conversations. . . . Analysis . . . involved the review of audio-tapes and verbatim transcripts of the tape-recorded interviews to get a general sense of the experience for each participant, to identify particular ideas within each account, and then to make connections among all of the participants' accounts. Final accounts or narratives are the interpretations made by members of the research team. . . . Discussion of our findings with colleagues . . . enriched understandings and pointed the way to further work that needs to be done" (p. 31).

(Excerpted and summarized from Mackinnon, McIntyre, and Quance 2005)

The Methods section delineates how the MacKinnon team collected their data. Note that investigators used interviews for data collection rather than quantitative measuring instruments. The Data Analysis section describes the process for conducting interviews. The Methods section also provides readers with an explanation of the interview process. This article does not specifically address methods to increase trustworthiness of data collection and analysis, although readers might infer some of these elements in the discussion of the analysis process. For example, the researchers indicate that they discussed their findings with colleagues, which *"enriched understandings and pointed the way to further work that needs to be done"* (MacKinnon et al. 2005, p. 31).

Finally, the segment on data analysis offers a stepped process for examining the interviews and deriving the themes of the study, including reviewing the tapes, transcribing them verbatim, making connections among them, and writing interpretive accounts of the interviews.

Applying the "examine" step of the SEE process will help you to identify specific segments of the article that reveal the investigator's methods of study. This information should provide you with a clearer picture of how researchers conduct studies and allow further reader examination to determine if sound research methods are used.

RESULTS. Now that we have examined the Introduction and Methods sections, we will address the Results section. This section presents a more detailed picture of the study participants and provides answers to the questions raised in the introduction. Figure 8-4 offers criteria for examining study findings or results. Characteristics of study participants provide a more complete picture of the sample. Findings explain the answers to the research questions or hypotheses and look quite different for quantitative and qualitative studies. In quantitative studies, statistical significance informs you of any differences or relationships that were found. The narrative picture painted in qualitative studies share what the data revealed.

When you examine the Results section of the Schoenfelder and Rubenstein article (see Box 8-7), you will easily find the description of the study participants under a

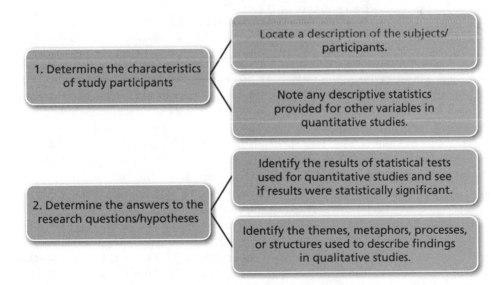

■ FIGURE 8-4 Process for Examining the Results Section
Systematically reading the results answers the questions raised in the study's introduction.

> ### BOX 8-7 Excerpts from Results Section of Quantitative Article
>
> **Sample Characteristics**
> "The initial sample ($N = 81$) consisted of 62 women and 19 men between the ages of 64 and 100 years (mean = 84.1). The demographic, mobility, and activity characteristics for the entire sample at pretest are summarized in Table 1. Fifty-three percent of the participants had fallen in the past year. Baseline mean scores for selected sample characteristics and fall-related variables are reported in Table 2. There were no significant baseline differences between the intervention and control groups for all outcome measures" (p. 25).
>
> **Study Results**
> "Mobility status at baseline was significantly associated with balance, walking time, falls efficacy, and risk of falling (chi-square p values < .05). Because of this association, all group and repeated measures analyses controlled for baseline mobility. Mobility status was significantly associated with age but not gender. The mean age for independent walkers was 5 to 7 years younger than the mean ages for the assistance groups. . . . Most elders were able to complete the parallel stance for 10 seconds at baseline, and there was no significant change within or between groups over time. Among those who used assistive devices and for all mobility levels combined, a significantly larger proportion of the intervention group showed maintenance or improvement over time with the semi-tandem stance compared with the control group at the completion of the exercise program at 3 months. This finding also remained significant at 6 months, even though the intervention group had not done the supervised exercise program for 3 months. In the time period from 3 to 6 months, among those who used an assistive device, a significantly larger proportion of the intervention group exhibited the same or improvement in fear of falling compared with the control group. Most other outcome variables exhibited nonsignificant changes over time in the predicted direction (indicated in bold in Table 3). Lack of significance was most likely related to the small numbers of respondents in each mobility group" (pp. 26–27).
>
> (Excerpted from Schoenfelder and Rubenstein 2004)

subhead appropriately entitled "Sample Characteristics". The verbal description is quite clear, and accompanying tables (which we do not reproduce here) offer additional detail about the reported variables. When examining a study to determine answers to the research questions/hypotheses, remind yourself of what those questions or hypotheses are. Recall from your examination of the Introduction (see page 169) that the Schoenfelder team's hypothesis was: ". . . *the proportion of elders with consistent or improved fall-related outcomes would be significantly higher for those individuals participating in the ankle-strengthening and walking program than for those elders who did not participate.*" An examination of the excerpt reveals that: ". . . *those who used assistive devices and for all mobility levels combined, a significantly larger proportion of the intervention group showed maintenance or improvement overtime with the semi-tandem stance . . . at 3 months.*" See Box 8-7 for additional findings that indicate the finding was stable over time ("*6 months . . .*"), and that those receiving the intervention exhibited either the same or improved levels of fear of falling. Find the statement in Box 8-7 that speaks to the outcome of the other variables measured (Schoenfelder and Rubenstein 2004, pp. 25–26).

The Results section from the MacKinnon et al. (2005) qualitative study included in Box 8-8 looks and feels very different from the quantitative study's results. The description

BOX 8-8 Excerpts from Results Section of Qualitative Study

"Analysis of the in-depth interviews suggests that women attribute multiple meanings to the care provided by labor and delivery nurses . . . What stood out in each of these women's accounts . . . was that a nurse's presence was the way in which a nurse was "there" for them and was a very important part of their experience. One woman said: I went in know-ing . . . that the doctor wouldn't be around all the time, but I don't think you realize how much dependency you have on the nurses . . . (Nancy, first baby) . . ." (p. 32).

"Women also described the kind of nursing presence they needed during childbirth. Women wanted the nurse to be available, to be emotionally involved, to help create a special moment, to hear and respond to their concerns, to share the responsibility for keeping them safe, and to act as a "go-between" for their family and the medical institution. Janet . . . described the nurse as someone who has seen the whole process and knows the experience, who can an-ticipate your needs and be a "little bit more emotionally involved, . . ." (p. 32).

"The women's experience was greatly enhanced by having the opportunity to get to know the nurse and by feeling that the nurse knew them . . . This feeling of being known and un-derstood was enhanced when nurses provided information about what was happening and kept the woman informed and involved as her labor progressed. Sarah (first baby) said, "I was quite concerned about that and, you know, about the possibility of decisions being made on my behalf and it being explained to me afterwards . . ." Knowing the woman was understood as [nurses] recognizing the uniqueness of her [mother's] situation . . ." (p. 32).

"Another important finding from our study was that women wanted the opportunity to get to know the nurses who cared for them. Needing to know and trust their nurse became a more pressing concern for these women as labor advanced and women drew inward to do the work of labor . . . Another woman (Teresa, second baby) described needing to 'let go' of some of her responsibility as her labor progressed and needing to share this responsibility with a known and trusted nurse" (p. 32).

"Our analysis of these women's accounts suggested that women's experiences of a nurse's presence and the meanings attributed to them cannot be understood apart from the insti-tutional structures and processes that shape them. For example . . . Women in our study described triage as a "holding tank" where routine procedures were carried out and "the forms" completed. Women felt powerless as they waited for the doctor, felt they were not heard, and felt their experiences of labor were invalidated" (p. 33).

"Our research clearly demonstrated that women value the support work of labor and de-livery nurses. Another finding from this exploratory study was that the labor and delivery nurse's role is very complex; relationships must be established and trust built under difficult circumstances. . . . The practice of skilled labor and delivery nurses is highly individualized, contextual, and reflective. Intrapartum nursing practice, then, is a complex art that can be experienced as a call for nursing presence" (p. 33).

(Excerpted from MacKinnon et al. 2005)

is entirely narrative and includes no statistical or numerical measures. To ascertain some of the participants' characteristics, readers must look back to the Participants and Setting discussed in the Methods section. This section described ages and time since birth. The number of births (*first baby versus second baby*) provides further description in the Results section (MacKinnon et al. 2005, p. 32).

Looking back to the Introduction reminds us that the purpose of the study was *"to develop new understandings of what it means for a nurse to be present during childbirth."* While there are no numbers used in qualitative studies, descriptions detailing categories of importance and care reveal the answers to the study purpose. For example *". . . [nurse's] presence was an important part of their experience; women wanted the nurse to be available, to be emotionally involved, to help create a special moment."* Additionally, *"...women's experience was greatly enhanced by having the opportunity to get to know the nurse and by feeling that the nurse knew them . . ."* and *". . . women wanted the opportunity to get to know the nurses who cared for them"*. Findings also indicate that institutional structures and processes played a role in women's experiences of nurses' presence. Findings further indicate that women valued the support of labor and delivery nurses. Notice that direct quotes from participants provide examples of the aspect of the described phenomenon of nurse presence. These quotes serve the function that numbers serve in quantitative studies. (Example: *"Janet . . . described the nurse as someone who has seen the whole process and knows the experience, who can anticipate your needs and be a "little bit more emotionally involved, . . ."*) See if you can find other examples of direct participant quotes in this section. The researchers' description, supported by the quotes, provides a picture of the phenomenon of nurse presence during labor and delivery (MacKinnon et al. 2005, pp. 32–33).

DISCUSSION OR CONCLUSIONS. Last, you should examine the study's Discussion section. Figure 8-5 offers guidelines for examining a study's discussion and conclusions. This section helps to elaborate on how to interpret the findings and examine how findings relate to previously published literature. Implications of the findings illustrate how to improve nursing practices and also share any factors that might limit how we may apply the findings.

Box 8-9 contains discussion excerpts from the quantitative article and Box 8-10 contains excerpts from the qualitative article.

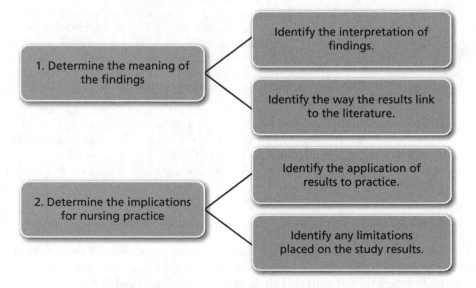

■ **FIGURE 8-5** Critically reading the Discussion section helps you to interpret the researcher's findings and understand their implications.

BOX 8-9 Discussion Excerpts from Quantitative Study

"There were significant changes as hypothesized for semi-tandem stance. The exercise program emphasized balance and did indeed improve balance as measured by the semi-tandem stance. Not only was balance maintained or improved at the completion of the supervised exercise program, the effect remained significant 3 months after completion of the program. This finding suggests that interruption in an exercise program does not mean the positive effects are immediately lost. Reestablishing the exercise program after an illness or injury or hospitalization would therefore be warranted for elderly nursing home residents. The tandem stance was too difficult for most subjects to do and therefore did not show significant maintenance or improvement . . ." (p. 27).

"It was expected that ankle strength would be significantly affected by the exercise program because there was an exercise specifically targeted at strengthening ankles. Although the results were not significant, the results for all mobility levels were in the predicted direction ($p = .08$) . . . Lower strength gain (knees and ankles) was significantly associated with increase in gait speed and improved falls efficacy (Chandler, Duncan, Kochersberger, and Studenski, 1998), two of the fall-related outcomes in this study. . . . Recent findings suggest that interventions for increasing ankle ROM may increase balance and reduce falls in older adults (Mecagni, Smith, Roberts, and O'Sullivan, 2000) . . ." (pp. 28–29).

"Major strengths of this study were the use of a control group, excellent adherence to the exercise program and no reported adverse effects to the exercise program . . . There were limitations with this research. . . . Recruitment was somewhat difficult in that some potential subjects were hesitant to start an exercise program. Attrition was also a limitation in this study that reduced the sample size to 67 at the 3-month follow-up and to 58 at the 6-month follow-up. . . ." (p. 29).

"The findings in this study have implications for nursing research. The results show promise that a simple exercise plan can have positive effects on fall-related outcomes, especially balance and fear of falling as indicated by this study . . . Recommendations can be made for nursing practice based on this research. Nursing home staff can easily be trained to use the exercise program . . . Along with implementing the exercise program, walking in general should be emphasized   Interventions to decrease the chances of falling need to be identified through research efforts and applied in nursing practice. There is mounting evidence that exercise can improve fall-related outcomes for older adults, even frail elders . . . " (p. 29).

(Excerpted from Schoenfelder and Rubenstein 2004)

As we examine the excerpt in Box 8-9, we immediately find an interpretation of the findings in the first paragraph: "*The exercise program emphasized balance and did indeed improve balance as measured by the semi-tandem stance . . .* " (Schoenfelder and Rubenstein 2004, p. 27). This interpretation continues in the second paragraph, in the discussion of ankle strength and mobility levels. The citations of other literature in this paragraph clearly indicate instances where the results tied into existing research. The excerpt also makes a clear statement of study strengths and limitations in paragraph three. Paragraph four discusses the possible use of the results in nursing practice.

The MacKinnon et al. study's Discussion section found in Box 8-10 includes some key sentences that help to summarize the research and provide further interpretation of the findings. For example, the second paragraph begins: "*Women in this study*

BOX 8-10 Discussion Excerpts from Qualitative Study

"Future research is needed to explicate the institutional processes affecting the support work of intrapartum nurses. Although previous research has identified the benefits of supportive care in labor (Hodnett, 2002; Scot et al., 1999), other research suggests that nurses do not consistently provide supportive care (Gagnon and Waghorn, 1996; Gale et al., 2001; McNiven et al., 1992). Despite these findings, there has been little attempt to study those elements of the work place setting that affect the support work of labor and delivery nurses" (p. 33).

"Women in this study identified institutional structures (such as obstetric triage) and work processes (such as rules that structured the provision of nursing care) negatively affecting their childbearing experiences. Analysis of the data from our study suggests that women's experiences of a nurse's presence cannot be understood apart from the institutional structures and work processes that influence what the nurse can and cannot do. Institutional ethnography could be used as methodology to explicate the social and institutional determinants of intrapartum nursing practice" (Campbell and Gregor, 2002; DeVault and McCoy, 2002; Smith, 1987) (p. 33).

"The meaning of the nurse's presence for these women was based on a relationship and getting to know and trust their nurse. Rubin (1984) also found that women's trust in intrapartum nurses increased when women perceived nurses as well qualified and as understanding their unique situation and needs. . . . Knowing the woman and providing the opportunity for her to get to know and trust her nurse is very difficult to accomplish within existing institutional structures. . . ." (p. 34).

"Women in this study articulated that as labor advanced, so did their need to be able to trust their nurse(s) so that they could let go of some of the responsibility for the safety of their baby. Drawing on Rubin's work, Sleutel proposed that intrapartum nurses also need to be skilled at 'facilitating a woman's ability to totally surrender her body to a uniquely feminine task: that of giving birth' (2003, p. 77). The presence of a known and trusted nurse might provide women with the opportunity to let go of some of the responsibility and 'do' their primary job of labor. Skillful intrapartum nursing practice, then, requires both knowing what to do (knowing in general) and knowing about the particular concerns of this woman (contextual and situated knowing) . . . " (p. 34).

"Nurses need to ask themselves whether and how biomedical 'surveillance' can be accomplished in partnership with woman and families. Nurses need to be aware that technical functions and 'nursing the chart' to reduce legal liability may conflict with their support work, leaving women feeling alone and abandoned" (p. 34).

---

identified institutional structures (such as obstetric triage) and work processes (such as rules that structured the provision of nursing care) negatively affecting their childbearing experiences. . ."). The researchers expand on the finding that institutional structures and processes merge and influence women's experiences in labor and delivery. This idea results in a recommendation for further research and calls for an institutional ethnography to "*explicate the social and institutional determinants of intrapartum nursing practice.*" Other research ideas reveal ties to literature such as references regarding the "*benefits of supportive care during labor,*" and "*that nurses do not consistently provide supportive care.*" The MacKinnon team ends the Discussion section with a recommendation for applying their findings to practice (MacKinnon et al. 2005, pp. 33–34).

Evaluate

The final step in the SEE process is to **evaluate** the study. Evaluation involves making judgments about the value of the study and deciding whether the study is a good one. This process is commonly referred to as a **research critique**. It judges the theoretical and methodological merits of the study and addresses issues such as whether a study was theoretically sound, whether it was appropriately designed, and whether the methods or statistical analysis were correctly applied. These judgments require considerable knowledge of research and statistical methodologies. While you do not yet possess the knowledge or skills necessary to offer a critical evaluation of a reported research study, you will gain this expertise as you develop and practice as a nurse. As a novice research consumer you need to rely on research published in established professional journals. In this way, you depend on the editors and reviewers of the journal to make those critical evaluations about the theoretical and methodological merits of the study.

> **Consider This . . .**
>
> Do you ever feel a little queasy when asked to do an evaluation or make a judgment? What would make you feel more comfortable in evaluating studies?

However, there are questions that you can ask that have a bearing on the quality of the study. See Box 8-11 for a series of questions that you can ask about the quality of a quantitative research study.

Because of differences between quantitative and qualitative studies, readers need to ask different evaluative questions about qualitative studies. See Box 8-12 for suggestions regarding evaluation of qualitative studies.

One key concern when evaluating a study is whether you will be able to apply the results to a particular practice setting. In a quantitative study, the question is: *Are the results generalizable to subjects other than those in the study?* If you remember from Chapter 3, results are generalizable to the population when the researchers use probability sampling. If they did not, it is more difficult to generalize the findings to other groups. One strategy you can consider is whether other studies have generated similar results. If more than one study shows similar results, you can be more confident in their validity. If the researchers used a theoretical framework, that too might broaden the applicability of results to other groups of subjects.

While qualitative studies do not have the generalizability (transferability) of experimental studies, nonetheless readers do look at potential applicability to practice. The key question here is whether the results will be relevant to nursing practice (i.e., does the interpretation of the data and the resulting themes, patterns, structures, or processes include logically coherent ideas and advice on how they might be applied to the practice of nursing?).

Let's revisit our two articles in light of the checklists for evaluating research shown in Box 8-11 and Box 8-12. The article in which Schoenfelder's team presented their quantitative study on the effect of exercise on falls was solid. Key elements of the study were easy to identify and the steps of the research process were generally easy to follow. There was a clear and succinct presentation of key ideas. The introductory argument clearly states the researchers' primary purpose and their hypothesis. The hypothesis told us precisely what the researchers were trying to discover.

BOX 8-11 Checklist to Evaluate Quantitative Research Studies

	Yes	No
Title and Abstract		
Does title indicate nature of study?	_____	_____
Does abstract provide study overview?	_____	_____
Introduction or Background		
Were key elements of the study clearly identified?	_____	_____
Were research questions/hypotheses clearly stated and easily understood?	_____	_____
Do the researchers state a theoretical framework?	_____	_____
Methodology		
Were the steps of the research process easy to follow?	_____	_____
What sampling technique(s) were used?	_____	
	_____	
Were instruments reliable and valid?	_____	_____
Findings		
Were study questions clearly answered?	_____	_____
Discussion		
Were study findings tied back to existing knowledge?	_____	_____
Did the ideas presented make logical or intuitive sense?	_____	_____
Were results of similar studies reviewed in the article?	_____	_____
Were ideas concisely and comprehensively presented?	_____	_____
Overall Questions		
Are the results generalizable to subjects other than those in the study?	_____	_____
How similar is my practice setting to the study setting?	_____	_____
How similar are my patients to the subjects in the study?	_____	_____
Can I use these findings in my practice?	_____	_____

Subheadings in the Methods section clearly delineated key parts of the study methodology. Reliability and validity of multiple instruments were directly and comprehensively addressed. The Results section directly addressed the hypothesis and answered the identified research problem. Study findings made ties to existing knowledge. A convenience sampling technique means that the results are limited to the sample tested. There are also limits on applicability because of sample attrition and the use of a predominantly Caucasian sample from one state. However, these results are consistent with other study results that recommend exercise for the elderly. The trial use of a walking and ankle-strengthening program in a clinical practice setting such as a nursing home might prove to be a valuable intervention in reducing falls.

BOX 8-12 Evaluative Questions for Qualitative Research Studies

	Yes	No
Title and Abstract		
Does title indicate nature of study?	_____	_____
Does abstract provide study overview?	_____	_____
Introduction or Background		
Were key elements of the study clearly identified?	_____	_____
Were research questions or aims clearly stated and easily understood?	_____	_____
Are philosophical underpinnings identified?	_____	_____
Methodology		
Could you readily follow steps of the research process?	_____	_____
How was the sample obtained?	_____	
	_____	
What methods were used to gather data?	_____	
	_____	
How were data analyzed?	_____	
	_____	
Results/Findings		
Were the phenomena fully described?	_____	_____
Did the narrative paint a clear picture of the phenomenon?	_____	_____
Were themes, structures, or processes clearly presented?	_____	_____
Did these themes, structures, or processes make sense?	_____	_____
Could you see how the themes, structures, or processes were supported by the data as evidenced by participant quotes?	_____	_____
Discussion		
Were study findings tied back to existing knowledge?	_____	_____
Did the ideas presented make logical or intuitive sense?	_____	_____
Were results of similar studies reviewed in the article?	_____	_____
Were ideas concisely and comprehensively presented?	_____	_____
Overall Questions		
Are the results relevant to your particular practice?	_____	_____
Does the interpretation of the data and the resulting themes, patterns, structures, or processes make sense in your practice?	_____	_____
Are the findings useful?	_____	_____

The MacKinnon team's qualitative study also clearly identifies its elements and builds an argument for the usefulness of the study. The research question was clearly stated in its own titled section of the article. Researchers identified using hermeneutic phenomenology and briefly discussed how they applied the philosophical underpinnings. Researchers laid out the study process. Qualitative studies have limitations in generalizability or transferability of findings to other groups. For example, investigators used purposive sampling techniques to obtain the six participants. It is difficult to know the degree to which participants selected through this process represent all women undergoing labor and delivery. While these six participants may have offered in-depth descriptions of their experiences, it is difficult to discern if the labor and delivery patients in this study are similar to those that might be found in other practices. The study occurred in Canada, a country with universal health insurance coverage. Are these participants and the labor and delivery services they had access to similar to those found in a rural Texas town or the teaching hospital of a major U.S. city? There is not enough information to be certain.

However, the researchers' descriptions of the phenomenon make sense and the data support them. Quotes from study participants further support the researchers' interpretation. Labor and delivery nurses or other mothers who have recently delivered babies may find that their experiences closely match findings of this study. Another strength of this study is that its findings are compared to those of the theorist Rubin (1984) and other researchers (Example: Hodnett 2002; Scot et al. 1999; and several others—see citations in discussion). That the MacKinnon team's study outcomes were congruent with those of previously conducted studies lends weight to their credibility.

Health care research carries currency not only in the health care world where it is conducted, but also in the popular press. Consider the *Research in the News* box that contains a summary and discussion of research findings regarding a ground-breaking mammography study. A synopsis of the news article run in the *New York Times* is included. This article will be contrasted with the abstract of the actual study from the *New England Journal of Medicine*.

Research in the News: Part 1

Mammograms' Value in Cancer Fight at Issue

BY GINA KOLATA
New York Times, September 23, 2010,
On Page A1

A new study suggests that increased awareness and improved treatments rather than mammograms are the main force in reducing the breast cancer death rate.

Starting in their 40s or 50s, most women in this country faithfully get a mammogram every year, as recommended by health officials. But the study suggests that the decision about whether to have the screening test may now be a close call.

The study, medical experts say, is the first to assess the benefit of mammography in the context of the modern era of breast cancer treatment. While it is unlikely to settle the debate over mammograms—and experts continue to disagree about the value of the test—it indicates that improved treatments with hormonal therapy and other targeted drugs may have, in a way, washed out most of mammography's benefits by making it less important to find cancers when they are too small to feel.

Previous studies of mammograms, done decades ago, found they reduced the breast cancer death rate by 15 to 25 percent, a meaningful amount. But that was when treatment was much less effective.

In the new study, mammograms, combined with modern treatment, reduced the death rate by 10 percent, but the study data indicated that the effect of mammograms alone could be as low as 2 percent or even zero. A 10 percent reduction would mean that if 1,000 50-year-old women were screened over a decade, 996 women rather than 995.6 would not die from the cancer—an effect so tiny it may have occurred by chance.

The study, published Thursday in the New England Journal of Medicine, looked at what happened in Norway before and after 1996, when the country began rolling out mammograms for women ages 50 to 69 along with special breast cancer teams to treat all women with breast cancer.

The study is not perfect. The ideal study would randomly assign women to have mammograms or not. But, cancer experts said, no one would do such a study today when mammograms are generally agreed to prevent breast cancer deaths. In the study, which is continuing, women were followed for a maximum of 8.9 years. It is possible that benefits may emerge later.

Nonetheless, the new study is "very credible," said Dr. Barnett Kramer, associate director for disease prevention at the National Institutes of Health.

"This is the first time researchers used real populations to compare the effects of treatment and mammography in the modern era of treatment," Dr. Kramer said. "It shows the relative impacts of screening versus therapy in an era in which therapy has been improving. . . ."

In their study, the investigators analyzed data from all 40,075 Norwegian women who had received a diagnosis of breast cancer from 1986 to 2005, a time when treatment was changing markedly.

In that period, 4,791 women died. And, starting in 1996, Norway began offering mammograms to women ages 50 to 69 and assigning multidisciplinary treatment teams to all women with breast cancer, similar to the teams at many major medical centers in the United States. The question was, Did the program of mammograms and optimal new treatment with coordinated teams of surgeons, pathologists, oncologists, radiologists and nurses lower the breast cancer death rate?

The investigators found that women 50 to 69 who had mammograms and were treated by the special teams had a 10 percent lower breast cancer death rate than similar women who had had neither.

They also found, though, that the death rate fell by 8 percent in women over 70 who had the new treatment teams but had not been invited to have

continued . . .

mammograms. And Dr. Kramer said he knew of no evidence that breast cancer was more easily treated in women over 70 than in women ages 50 to 69.

That means, Dr. H. Gilbert Welch of Dartmouth wrote in an additional analysis in an accompanying editorial, that mammography could have reduced the breast cancer death rate by as little as 2 percent, an amount so small that it is not really different from zero.

...

Dr. Laura Esserman, a professor of surgery and radiology at the University of California in San Francisco, said it tells her that "if you get the same treatment and the outcome is the same if you find it earlier or later, then you don't make a difference when you find it early."

And screening has a cost, Dr. Welch said. Screening 2,500 50-year-olds for a decade would identify 1,000 women with at least one suspicious mammogram resulting in follow-up tests. Five hundred would have biopsies. And 5 to 15 of those women would be treated for cancers that, if left alone, would have grown so slowly they would never have been noticed.

When the study was planned, the scientists expected that screening would be even more effective than it was in studies from decades ago. After all, mammography had improved and, in Norway, each mammogram was independently read by two radiologists, which should make it less likely that cancers would be missed. The researchers expected mammograms to reduce the breast cancer death rate by a third. . . .

Marvin Zelen, a statistician at the Harvard School of Public Health and the Dana-Farber Cancer Institute, who was a member of the research team said even though the mammography benefit is small, if he were a woman he would get screened.

"It all depends on how you approach risk," Dr. Zelen said. His approach, he says, is "minimax"—he wants to minimize the maximum risk—which, in this case, is dying of a cancer.

Dr. Kalager came to the opposite conclusion. She worries about the small chance of benefit in light of the larger chance of finding and treating a cancer that did not need to be treated. . . .

Read the headline news report concerning mammography. This report challenges prior thinking about the value of mammograms.

- What shift in current mammography practice is proposed?

   A key sentence explaining the rationale for shifts in thinking regarding mammography is

   . . . it indicates that improved treatments with hormonal therapy and other targeted drugs may have, in a way, washed out most of mammography's benefits by making it less important to find cancers when they are too small to feel.

   This sentence tells us that a key factor, improved treatment modalities, has shifted the effect that mammograms have on long term survival.

- What are some of the study limitations discussed that might influence study findings? Note the following:
  - No random assignment of women to groups. This means that the comparison groups may not have been equal to begin with.
  - Time length of study may not have been long enough to discover future benefits.
- Does everyone agree about the implications of the study findings? What should the public believe?

Check out the news story at:

http://www.nytimes.com/2010/09/23/health/research/23mammogram.html

Resource and Subject Matter

Research in the News: Part 2

Effect of Screening Mammography on Breast-Cancer Mortality in Norway

KALAGER, M., ZELEN, M., LANGMARK, F., AND ADAMI, H.
N Engl J Med 2010; 363:1203–1210, September 23, 2010

Background: A challenge in quantifying the effect of screening mammography on breast-cancer mortality is to provide valid comparison groups. The use of historical control subjects does not take into account chronologic trends associated with advances in breast-cancer awareness and treatment.

Methods: The Norwegian breast-cancer screening program was started in 1996 and expanded geographically during the subsequent 9 years. Women between the ages of 50 and 69 years were offered screening mammography every 2 years. We compared the incidence-based rates of death from breast cancer in four groups: two groups of women who from 1996 through 2005 were living in counties with screening (screening group) or without screening (nonscreening group); and two historical-comparison groups that from 1986 through 1995 mirrored the current groups.

Results: We analyzed data from 40,075 women with breast cancer. The rate of death was reduced by 7.2 deaths per 100,000 person-years in the screening group as compared with the historical screening group (rate ratio, 0.72; 95% confidence interval [CI], 0.63 to 0.81) and by 4.8 deaths per 100,000 person-years in the nonscreening group as compared with the historical nonscreening group (rate ratio, 0.82; 95% CI, 0.71 to 0.93; P<0.001 for both comparisons), for a relative reduction in mortality of 10% in the screening group (P=0.13). Thus, the difference in the reduction in mortality between the current and historical groups that could be attributed to screening alone was 2.4 deaths per 100,000 person-years, or a third of the total reduction of 7.2 deaths.

Conclusions: The availability of screening mammography was associated with

continued . . .

a reduction in the rate of death from breast cancer, but the screening itself accounted for only about a third of the total reduction. *(Funded by the Cancer Registry of Norway and the Research Council of Norway.)*

Compare this *New England Journal of Medicine* abstract regarding the mammography study to the article excerpt on mammography from the *New York Times.*

- How does the information in this abstract differ from the information in the news article? Note:
  - Level of study detail, especially the findings
  - Specific conclusions of study
- What are possible reasons why the level of information and discussion of study conclusions are managed differently between the professional and lay press?
  - Is the public sufficiently informed regarding the study outcomes? Why or why not?

View the entire article at:

Kalager, M., M. Zelen, F. Langmark, and H. Adami. 2010. Effect of screening mammography on breast cancer mortality in Norway. *New England Journal of Medicine, 363*: 1203-1210.

Resource and Subject Matter

SUMMARY

In this chapter, you have learned about the structure and format of published research articles, reviewed a mechanism for critically reading those articles, and walked through that critical reading process using two sample articles. Key points discussed in this chapter include the following:

- Many research articles use standard elements to present a study. Components include (a) the title and abstract, (b) introduction and background, (c) methods, (d) results or findings, (e) discussion or conclusions, and (f) references. *(Objective 1)*

- Each element of a journal article has a specific function that reflects aspects of the research process.
  - The **TITLE** describes the study while the **Abstract** provides an overview of the study process and findings.
  - The **Introduction and Background** section includes the problem statement or purpose, literature review, theoretical framework, and the hypotheses or research questions; alternatively, it may simply state the study objective or aims.
  - The **Methods** section discusses research design, sample and setting, data collection procedures, and data analysis procedures.
  - The **Results** or **Findings** section describes the sample and the study outcomes.
  - The **Discussion** or **Conclusions** section is where researchers interpret study results, make recommendations for further research, and discuss implications for nursing.
  - Finally, the **References** section includes full citations for all sources used in the article. *(Objective 2)*

- The SEE (Scan, Examine, Evaluate) process is a **critical reading** strategy that helps you determine whether an article's findings will be applicable to nursing practice. *(Objective 3)*

- The first step of the SEE process is to **survey** the article, scanning it for a general understanding of its purpose and direction. You can glean a lot of information about an article by checking its title, reading the abstract, and skimming the text and references. *(Objective 4)*

- Next, **examine** the article section by section to gain a better understanding of the researcher's study. Read the introduction to discover more about the study problem and its context; find the problem statement, hypothesis, or research question; ascertain the researchers' rationale for conducting the study; see if the literature review ties the research to the existing body of knowledge; and see if the study has a theoretical framework. Read the Methods discussion to determine how the study was conducted, including the research design, sample, setting, data collection techniques, variables under study, information about reliability and validity, and data analysis procedures. Read the Results section to find the answers to the research question/hypothesis stated in the Introduction. Read the Discussion section to find the researchers' interpretation of the results and their implications for nursing practice. Determine whether the researchers identify limitations to their findings. *(Objective 5)*

- The final step of the SEE process is to **evaluate** the study to determine its quality and validity. To do so, experienced nurse researchers conduct what is called a **research critique**. They use targeted questions, often in the form of a checklist, to systematically examine a research study in order to determine its usefulness. The checklists help nurse researchers assess the study for its theoretical and methodological merits. *(Objective 6)*

STUDENT ACTIVITIES

Now it is time for you to see whether you can apply what you have learned about systematically reading research. Work the exercises designed for this chapter.

1. Here is a list of study titles (each title is printed in blue). Based on the study title, classify the study as either quantitative or qualitative. What characteristics of the title helped you to decide what kind of study it was?

   a. Barnason, S., L. Zimmerman, M. Hertzog, and P. Schulz. 2010. Pilot testing of a medication self-management transition intervention for heart failure patients. *Western Journal of Nursing Research, 32*: 849.

   b. Deitrick, L., J. Bokovoy, and A. Panik. 2010. The "dance" continues . . . evaluating differences in call bell use between patients in private rooms and patients in double rooms using ethnography. *Journal of Nursing Care Quality,* 25(4): 279–287.

   c. Evans, M.J. and C.E. Hallett. 2007. Living with dying: A hermeneutic phenomenological study of the work of hospice nurses. *Journal of Clinical Nursing, 16*(4): 742–751.

d. Howard, V.M., C. Ross, A.M. Mitchell, and G.M. Nelson. 2010. "Human patient simulators and interactive case studies: a comparative analysis of learning outcomes and student perceptions." *CIN: Computer, Informatics, Nursing, 28*(1): 42–48.

e. Walker, S.N., C.H. Pullen, P.A. Hageman, L.S. Boeckner, M. Hertzog, M.K. Oberdorfer, and M.J. Rutledge. 2010. Maintenance of activity and eating change after a clinical trial of tailored newsletters with older rural women. *Nursing Research, 59*(5): 311–321.

f. Tobin, G.A. and C. Begley. 2008. Receiving bad news: a phenomenological exploration of the lived experience of receiving a cancer diagnosis. *Cancer Nursing, 31*(5): E31–39.

g. Clarke, A., R. Sohanpal, G. Wilson, and S. Taylor. 2010. Patients' perceptions of early supported discharge for chronic obstructive pulmonary disease: A qualitative study. *Quality & Safety in Health Care, 19*(2): 95–98.

h. Matos, P., L. Neushotz, M. Griffin, and J. Fitzpatrick. 2010. An exploratory study of resilience and job satisfaction among psychiatric nurses working in inpatient units. *International Journal of Mental Health Nursing, 19*(5): 307–312.

2. This exercise will give you practice using information from a research abstract. Read the following abstract and respond to the questions at the end of the abstract.

Purpose: While nursing programs incorporate ethics and ethical decision making in the curricula, many nurses feel unprepared for ethical dilemmas encountered in practice. This sense of being poorly equipped can extend into practice despite substantial clinical expertise gained throughout careers.

The aim of this qualitative study was to gain insight into how mid-career nurses define and respond to ethical dilemmas.

Method: Fifteen midcareer nurse leaders in the Southwestern United States participated in focus group discussions regarding their experiences with ethical dilemmas in nursing practice. Focus group activities used a series of qualitative-based, iterative exercises designed to encourage dialogue about how mid-career nurses defined and responded to ethical dilemmas and the obstacles that existed in dilemma resolution. Recorders for each group kept a record of the discussions that were later transcribed, compiled, and analyzed.

Findings: Ranging in age from their mid-30s to late 50s, these well-seasoned, mid-career nurses functioned in practice roles as clinical specialists, nurse practitioners, nursing service administrators, and nursing educators. Mid-career nurses characterized ethical dilemmas as "the ones you never forget," charged with emotional intensity and conflict. Participants viewed ethical dilemmas differently than other practice problems, noting there was "no oracle to go to" for answers. While mid-career nurses were able to draw on a greater number of resources for dilemma resolution, they still felt considerable anguish.

Conclusions: Although mid-career nurses identified ethical dilemmas similar to those of less experienced nurses, they possessed more sophisticated mechanisms for resolution. However, dilemmas possessed a gut-wrenching emotional impact that made some nurses consider leaving nursing positions. Nurses perceived information-seeking and dialogue as effective methods for approaching dilemma resolution.

- What was the purpose for the study?
- Who composed the sample?
- How were data collected and analyzed?
- What were the major findings?
- Did this abstract give you sufficient information to help you decide whether to look up the entire article? Why or why not?

3. Use the SEE method to read the quantitative article and the qualitative article listed below. Remember these key points
   - Survey the entire article.
   - Examine the article components
     - Title and Abstract
     - Introduction and Background
     - Methods
     - Results or Findings
     - Discussion/Conclusions
   - Evaluate the quality of what you have read. Use the checklists in Boxes 8-11 and 8-12.

Read the quantitative article by Ganz, F., N. Fink, O. Raanan, M. Asher, M. Bruttin, M. Nun, and J. Benbinishty. 2009. ICU Nurses' oral-care practices and the current best evidence. *Journal of Nursing Scholarship, 41*(2): 132–138.

Read the qualitative article by Greco, K., L. Nail, J. Kendall, J. Cartwright, and D. Messecar. 2010. Mammography decision making in older women with a breast cancer family history. *Journal of Nursing Scholarship, 42*(3): 348–356.

(Responses to Questions 1 and 2)

1. **Study Titles**
   a. Quantitative
   b. Qualitative
   c. Qualitative
   d. Quantitative
   e. Quantitative
   f. Qualitative
   g. Qualitative
   h. Quantitative

2. **Study Titles**
   - What was the purpose for the study?
     To gain insight into how mid-career nurses define and respond to ethical dilemmas.
   - Who composed the sample?
     Fifteen mid-career nurses (may add additional information regarding age and professional roles).

- How were data collected and analyzed?

  Data were collected through focus groups that guided participants through a structured process to elicit study information. Recorders logged the information which was later compiled. Specific analytic steps not included.

- What were the major findings?

  Midcareer nurses experienced ethical dilemmas similar to less experienced nurses but used more effective mechanisms for resolution. Information and dialogue were perceived as viable mechanisms to facilitate dilemma resolution. Dilemmas were gut-wrenching.

- Did this abstract give you sufficient information to decide to look up the entire article? Why or why not?

  Student response and rationale.

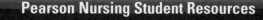

Pearson Nursing Student Resources

Find additional review materials at

www.nursing.pearsonhighered.com

Prepare for success with additional NCLEX®-style practice questions, interactive assignments and activities, web links, animations and videos, and more!

REFERENCES

deWitt, L., J. Ploeg, and M. Black. 2010. Living alone with dementia: An interpretive phenomenological study with older women. *Journal of Advanced Nursing, 66*(8): 1698–1707.

Doherty, M.E. 2010. Voices of midwives: A tapestry of challenges and blessings. *MCN: The American Journal of Maternal Child Nursing, 35*(2): 96–101.

El-Masri, M.M., S.M. Fox-Wasylyshyn, and T.A. Hammad. 2005. Predicting nosocomial bloodstream infections using surrogate markers of injury severity. *Nursing Research, 54*(4): 273–279.

Garcia, C. and E. Saewyc. 2007. Perceptions of mental health among recently immigrated Mexican adolescents. *Issues in Mental Health Nursing, 28:* 37–54.

Good, M., J. Gilbert, G. Anderson, S. Wotman, X. Cong, D. Lane, and S. Ahn. 2010. Supplementing relaxation and music for pain after surgery. *Nursing Research, 59*(4): 259–269.

Greco, K., L. Nail, J. Kendall, J. Cartwright, and D. Messecar. 2010. Mammography decision making in older women with a breast cancer family history. *Journal of Nursing Scholarship, 42*(3): 348–356.

MacKinnon, K., M. McIntyre, and M. Quance. 2005. The meaning of the nurse's presence during childbirth. *Journal of Obstetric, Gynecologic, and Neonatal Nursing, 34*(3): 28–36.

Newhouse, R.P., M. Johantgen, P.J. Pronovost, and E. Johnson. 2005. Perioperative nurses and patient outcomes-mortality, complications, and length of stay. *AORN Journal, 81*(3): 508–509, 513–516, 518, 520–522, 525–528.

Peterson, J.A., B.C. Yates, J.R. Atwood, and M. Hertzog. 2005. Effects of a physical activity intervention for women. *Western Journal of Nursing Research, 27*(1): 93–110.

Schoenfelder, D.P. and L.M. Rubenstein. 2004. An exercise program to improve fall-related outcomes in elderly nursing home residents. *Applied Nursing Research, 17*(1): 21–31.

Answer Key: The quantitative studies in **Box 8-1** are: El-Masri et al. (2005); Good et al. (2010); Newhouse et al. (2005); Peterson et al. (2005); Schoenfelder and Rubenstein (2004).

Appraising Evidence for Practice

CHAPTER OBJECTIVES

1. Compare and contrast the concepts of research utilization and evidence-based practice in nursing.
2. Identify EBP models that can be used to facilitate evidence in nursing practice.
3. Discuss types of resources used to produce evidence for practice.
4. Describe the use of evidence hierarchies to grade and recommend evidence for practice.
5. Explain a five step process that can be used to examine clinical questions.
6. Apply the PICO(T) format in formulating clinical questions.
7. Analyze the process of locating, appraising, incorporating, and disseminating evidence in practice.

KEY TERMS

Clinical practice guidelines **(p. 199)**

Critically appraised topics (CATs) **(p. 201)**

Evidence-based (EB) model **(p. 196)**

Evidence-based practice (EBP) **(p. 195)**

Evidence hierarchy **(p. 201)**

Integrated research review (IRR) **(p. 198)**

Meta-analysis **(p. 199)**

Metasynthesis **(p. 199)**

PICO(T) **(p. 204)**

Research utilization **(p. 195)**

Systematic research review (SRR) **(p. 198)**

Systematic review **(p. 198)**

ABSTRACT

An evidence-based practice is based on the conscious effort to use research-based information in making decisions about patient care. There are six key steps that guide evidence-based practice: 1) problem identification, 2) evidence collection, 3) evidence appraisal, 4) evidence integration and intervention implementation, 5) outcome evaluation, and 6) disseminate outcome. Precisely formulating the problem using a specified question format detailing the population, intervention, comparison, and outcome serves as a foundation for the other four steps. Collecting the evidence takes a systematic and comprehensive approach. Appraising the evidence requires examining and assessing the studies using key questions to grade the evidence. Integration and implementation depend on the support available. Outcomes are used to evaluate the implementation of any intervention. Dissemination of the outcomes is the final step.

The purpose of this chapter is to assist you in translating research evidence into practice. This is important because it allows you to lay a foundation for your practice that is based on the best knowledge and most up-to-date information available in the literature. This allows you as a practitioner to make decisions about the care you administer with a high degree of confidence. We have already covered the skills that you need to search for and find relevant materials in Chapter 2. We also explored a strategy for surveying, examining, and evaluating research literature in Chapter 8. Now we are going to focus on using these and other skills to identify clinical problems and to find, critically evaluate, and use the best evidence possible to provide answers to those clinical problems. One of the goals here is to place the emphasis on a systematic process that seeks out the best research-based evidence rather than relying on more traditional modes of knowing such as authority, intuition, and trial and error.

Evidence-Based Practice and Research Utilization

Evidence-based practice (EBP) and research utilization are tools that practicing nurses use to ensure that they are equipped to make the most informed decisions about patient care. Recall from Chapter 1 that **evidence-based practice (EBP)** is defined as "the conscientious, explicit and judicious use of theory-derived, research-based information in making decisions about patient care delivery to individuals or groups of patients and in consideration of individual needs and preferences" (Ingersoll 2000, p. 152). There are several important features of the definition.

- It emphasizes a deliberate and systematic problem-solving approach.
- It makes use of research-based materials on which to base decisions.
- It considers how the decisions fit individual patient needs and preferences.
- It acknowledges that clinical expertise is key to integrating decisions into a specified care setting.

While the concepts of EBP and research utilization are sometimes used interchangeably, they are in fact two distinct concepts. **Research utilization** typically refers to finding a practical use for findings from a research study or studies in the real world of nursing practice. The process starts with the research findings that were generated and seeks to find a practical application. This process is often lengthy, and the implementation of important research findings can take years to become standard practice.

Research utilization may be categorized and validated as conceptual, instrumental, or persuasive (Estabrooks 1999). When we use research results to alter our perspectives without any particular specified change in our practice behaviors, that is *conceptual utilization*. We use the findings to expand our knowledge base. These findings may provide evidence to confirm things that we know or provide rationale to support clinical protocols that are already in place. However, they do not lead to specific changes in patient interventions. In contrast, *instrumental utilization* means that there is a concrete application of the research findings. A particular research study serves as a basis to change nursing interventions. The changes come as a direct result of the research findings. In persuasive utilization, research findings are used as a tool to advocate for a certain practice or intervention. It might be used informally to convince colleagues to alter some aspect of their clinical practice, or formally to persuade an organization or institution to change a particular policy, procedure, or prevailing practice.

Research utilization in nursing emerged in the 1970s and 1980s and was fueled by the large perceived gap between nursing research and nursing practice. As a result, many basic level nursing education programs began to include nursing research courses as a part of the required curriculum. Nursing research itself began to focus more on studies that addressed clinical nursing problems. Formally funded programs were launched to increase research utilization in practice. Many hospitals and other health care institutions undertook research utilization projects in the 1980s and 1990s in an attempt to increase research utilization in the practice arena.

EBP expands the conceptualization of research utilization. It seeks to find, critically examine, and synthesize all of the available evidence about specifically defined clinical problems. It then integrates this evidence with the clinical expertise of the nurse to make decisions about patient care that take into account the individual patient needs and values. So while research utilization starts with the research and moves to seeking practical applications, EBP begins with a clinical problem and seeks research-based evidence to undergird clinical decision-making.

Consider This . . .

What differences do you see in the concepts of research utilization and evidence-based practice?

As the notion of the importance of a research-based practice took hold across nursing education, research, and practice arenas, and the EBP movement swept through the health care community, the seeds for the evidence-based nursing practice movement were born. The move from the more narrowly defined concept of research utilization to a more expanded and complex concept of EBP began in nursing in the 1990s. This movement was a natural next step in nursing's journey to ground nursing care decisions on solid evidence.

Evidence-Based Practice

This section will present an overview of evidence-based (EB) models, discuss resources for locating viable evidence, and describe types and levels of evidence. An **evidence-based (EB) model** is a graphic representation of a defined process for collecting, evaluating, and using evidence. Most importantly we will introduce and discuss a process for integrating evidence into clinical practice.

From Research Utilization to Evidence-Based Practice

A number of nursing models were formulated during the era of research utilization to provide a conceptual structure for the use of research findings in practice. Many of these grew out of formally funded research utilization projects. A number of these models have been extended and altered to provide frameworks for EBP. Thus, they provide a road map for designing and implementing an evidence-based project in a particular clinical practice setting. Some, such as the Stetler model, are designed to be used by the individual clinician while others, such as the IOWA model, are designed to use an organizational approach. You can see examples and descriptions of some of these models below.

STETLER MODEL OF RESEARCH UTILIZATION. This model originated in 1976 to bridge the gap between research dissemination and its use in clinical practice. It was designed to promote critical thinking about application of research in the clinical area by individual nurse clinicians, and includes five process phases:

1. Preparation—identification of purpose and focus of literature review.
2. Validation—confirmation that the research data is relevant and applicable.
3. Comparative evaluation/decision-making—determination that study findings are relevant to the patients being cared for; determination to use or not use the findings.

4. Translation/application—determinations about how findings are to be applied in practice.

5. Evaluation—determination of the impact of the application.

This model was formulated for use by the individual nurse. It has been updated and expanded to embrace the concept of EBP (Stetler 1976; Stetler 2001).

IOWA MODEL. This model originated in 1994 at University of Iowa to promote quality of care in organizational settings through the use of research findings. It emphasizes the importance of the involvement of every level of an organization for success and is linked with quality assurance. The IOWA model examines both problem-focused and knowledge-focused triggers to identify a topic to explore and focuses on three key decisions:

1. Is the topic a priority?

2. Is there a sufficient research base?

3. Is change appropriate for adaption in practice?

The model was revised in 2001 to incorporate EBP and the development of EBP guidelines (Titler et al. 1994; Titler et al. 2001).

ROSSWURM AND LARRABEE MODEL. This model was developed in 1999 as a model to facilitate a change to evidence-based practice. Its six cyclical steps are similar to the nursing process:

1. Assess need for change.

2. Link interventions and outcomes.

3. Synthesize the evidence.

4. Design the practice change.

5. Implement and evaluate the change.

6. Integrate and maintain the change (Rosswurm and Larrabee 1999).

ACE STAR MODEL OF KNOWLEDGE TRANSFORMATION. This model, commonly referred to as the ACE Star model, was developed in 2004 by the University of Texas San Antonio Academic Center for EBP. It was intentionally developed as a framework in which to organize EBP processes and produce knowledge transformation. It entails a five-step process which is organized in the shape of a five-pointed star.

1. Discovery—knowledge generation stage which entails the conduct of research.

2. Summary—search, translation, summarization, and distillation of the applicable research into useable evidence summaries.

3. Translation—conversion of evidence summaries into practice recommendations.

4. Integration—change of individual and organizational practices through formal and informal means.

5. Evaluation—appraisal of the impact of the implemented EBP on patient outcomes, and on efficacy, efficiency, and economic impact (Stevens 2004).

You can read more about the ACE Star model and see a representation of the star on their website at www.acestar.uthscsa.edu/acestar-model.asp.

Resource and Subject Matter

While all of the models for EBP and research utilization offer different approaches to translating research into practice, there are remarkable similarities across the various models. All the models provide a specified process to follow in producing evidence-based change in practice. All identify a problem, collect evidence to address the problem, critically examine that evidence, and then design, implement, and evaluate the substantiated change. We will examine these steps later in this chapter.

Resources

As interest in establishing an evidence-based practice has risen, so have the available resources to help support an evidence-based practice. We have already discussed individual research studies, and these are the basic elements in building evidence for practice. However, there are other resources to consider in addition to the findings from individual research studies. This is evidence that has already been selected, critically assessed, and summarized by experts, and includes various types of systematic research reviews, clinical practice guidelines, and other summary types.

SYSTEMATIC REVIEWS. EBP relies heavily on the ability to locate, critically appraise, and integrate the available research. A systematic review can do all that work for you. The primary goal of a **systematic review** is to use a precise and methodological approach to search for, compile, and analyze the findings from a number of research studies. A summary of the findings can take one of several forms. The three most common forms are known as: 1) integrative research reviews (IRR)/systematic research reviews (SRR), 2) meta-analysis, and 3) metasynthesis (Whittemore 2005). While these are similar, they do differ from one another.

> ### Consider This . . .
> Why might systematic reviews be considered a crucial tool in evidence-based practice?

An **integrated research review (IRR)** is a narrative summary of past research findings on a certain topic in which the reviewer uses an analytic reasoning process to produce logical conclusions across the studies reviewed. The scope of an IRR can be as broad or as narrow as the topic that is selected. A **systematic research review (SRR)** is similar to an IRR, except that the findings sought are focused on a specific clinical problem rather than a broader clinical topic. The focus and scope in an SRR is narrow. The terms for IRR and SRR are frequently used interchangeably.

> ### BOX 9-1 Example of IRR/SRR
>
> Vanderbloom (2007) conducted an integrative review to answer the question "Does music reduce anxiety during invasive procedures with procedural sedation?" Thirteen research studies from the past 10 years met the criteria for the review. All studies were experimental and had a control and music intervention group. The review revealed that "music may be effective in lowering blood pressure and reducing medication requirements" (p. 15). The evidence needs to be supplemented with additional research to obtain more conclusive results about the role of music in reducing anxiety during procedures.

> ## BOX 9-2 Example of a Meta-Analysis
>
> Zhou et al. (2008) conducted a meta-analysis to investigate the relationships between children, parents, and nurses on pain ratings. Twelve non-experimental correlation studies that were published between 1990 and 2007 were selected for the meta-analysis. They found that the parent's and nurse's perceptions of the child's pain is only moderately correlated to the child's perception of pain, and should be considered as an estimate of the child's pain—not as a substitute of the child's self-rating of pain.

A **meta-analysis** searches for quantitative research studies that are asking the same research question and using a similar research design. It then uses a statistical analytic technique to treat the findings from all the studies as if they came from one large study. This allows for a greater confidence in and generalizability of the findings across the studies.

A **metasynthesis** searches for qualitative research studies that are looking at the same research topic. It then integrates the information found across the studies and offers fresh interpretations. Some metasyntheses concentrate on offering a fuller summary of the results across the studies. Others offer a reinterpretation of the collected materials and may even formulate a new theoretical frame of reference for the topic under exploration.

Systematic reviews can be found in a number of sources. The Cochrane and Dare databases we mentioned in Chapter 2 are maintained by the Cochrane Collaboration and contain nearly 10,000 systematic reviews on a wide range of clinical practice topics. These reviews are subject to strict review guidelines and are updated regularly. They maintain a website that is easily accessed by entering the term *Cochrane Library* in your internet search engine.

The Agency for Healthcare Research (AHRQ) serves as another important resource for systematic reviews. Fourteen selected evidence-based practice centers across the United States produce evidence reports to improve the quality of clinical care. You can locate these evidence reports by going to www.ahrq.gov. Roll over *clinical information* and click on evidence-based practice, and then click on the topical index (A–Z). As of April 2012 there are 1,205 evidence reports available for a wide variety of clinical practice topics.

> ## BOX 9-3 Example of a Metasynthesis
>
> Yick (2008) explored and synthesized the themes from eight qualitative articles on the role of spirituality (religiosity) with 62 survivors of domestic abuse. Forty-plus themes were reduced to nine more overarching themes: "1) strength and resilience, 2) tension stemming from religious definition of family, 3) tension stemming from religious definition of gender role expectations, 4) spiritual vacuum, 5) reconstruction, 6) recouping spirit and self, 7) new interpretations of submission, 8) forgiveness as healing, and 9) giving back" (p. 1289).

CLINICAL PRACTICE GUIDELINES. **Clinical practice guidelines** provide specific recommendations for clinical practice and have been constructed by experts from the best available evidence on a specific topic. A diverse panel of experts typically work together as a team to formulate the guidelines. The panel may include clinicians, health care administrators, policy makers, and consumers. These guidelines are usually based on systematic reviews such as those we just explored above and can be very useful as decision-making

Resources and Subject Matter

> **BOX 9-4** Sample Clinical Practice Guideline
>
> Practice guidelines for Oral Health: Nursing Assessment and Interventions were developed and published in 2006 by the RNAO. The guidelines are targeted at vulnerable adult populations who need assistance in meeting oral hygiene needs. A 13-member panel reviewed the evidence and issued a number of evidence-based interventions and recommendations for oral care (www.rnao.org).

tools in your clinical practice. In fact, many health care institutions incorporate these guidelines into their policy and procedure manuals for direction of care.

Consider This . . .

How does a clinical practice guideline differ from a systematic review?

It can often be overwhelming to search for evidence-based clinical practice guidelines, as there is no single database that houses them. There are also a number of so-called clinical guidelines available that are not in fact based on research evidence. There are, however, a number of sources available to help you find existing clinical practice guidelines. Specific databases are designed for to search for practice guidelines. The most well-known and all-encompassing is the National Guidelines Clearinghouse (NGC). The NGC serves as a public resource for evidence-based guidelines that have been formulated to improve and standardize clinical practice. The NGC was created by the AHRQ in collaboration with the American Medical Association, but it has expanded its efforts and now provides information for a broad spectrum of health care professionals. Other potentially useful resources for locating practice guidelines can be found in Box 9-5.

ADDITIONAL EVIDENCE TYPES. There are other types of evidence in addition to SSRs, clinical practice guidelines, and original research articles. You can also find summaries or synopses of systematic reviews as well as summaries of individual research studies. Journals such

> **BOX 9-5** Additional Resources for Locating Clinical Practice Guidelines
>
> American Cancer Society www.cancer.org
> Association of Women's Health, Obstetric & Neonatal Nursing (AWHONN) www.awhonn.org
> National Association of Neonatal Nurses (NANN) www.nann.org
> National Institute for Clinical Excellence (NICE) www.nice.org.uk
> Oncology Nursing Society (ONS) www.ons.org
> Registered Nurses Association of Ontario (RNAO) www.rnao.org
> Scottish Intercollegiate Guidelines Network (SIGN) www.sign.ac.uk
> University of Iowa Gerontological Nursing Interventions Research Center (GNIRC)
>   www.nursing.uiowa.edu/excellence/nursing_interventions/index.htm

as *Evidence-Based Nursing (EBN)* and *World Views on Evidence-Based Nursing* offer such summaries. EBN is offered online by subscription at http://ebn.bmj.com. It is probably also available through your library. *World Views on Evidence-Based Nursing* is published in association with Sigma Theta Tau International and offers an evidence digest feature that summarizes recent research. *Medscape Nurses*, sponsored by the National Institute for Nursing Research, offers monthly summaries of current nursing research and can be found online at www.medscape.com. *The Annual Review of Nursing Research*, which was discussed in Chapter 2, is an excellent resource for summaries of relevant research on selected topics.

   Critically appraised topics (CATs) and best practice information sheets are also available. CATs are currently featured primarily in medicine and feature a quick summary of the available key evidence for a particular clinical question with the clinical bottom line for practice succinctly spelled out. A number of resources are available online for various CATs. Just enter "critically appraised topics" in your internet search engine. A similar approach is found for a broader range of health care professionals in best practice information sheets offered by the Joanna Briggs Institute in Australia. These offer a summary of the available evidence, graded recommendations, and implications for practice for a variety of clinical issues. The information sheets are easily accessed at www.joannabriggs.edu.au.

Evidence Hierarchies

We have described a number of types of evidence and discussed the resources that help you locate these evidence types. So a new question might be how to sort out all these types of evidence. Fortunately there are tools to help do that. They are known as evidence hierarchies. There are a number of evidence hierarchies available. Most of the first evidence hierarchies were very medically oriented and relied heavily on the evidence produced by a particular kind of experimental research known as a randomized controlled trial. While this works well for certain medical interventions, it proved less than satisfactory for nursing and other types of health care practices. As the evidence-based practice movement has grown and spread to other areas of health care and other health care professionals, the guidelines for evidence have also evolved. The evidence hierarchy presented in Box 9-6 shows a generic evidence hierarchy that encompasses a fairly broad view of available evidence.

BOX 9-6 Evidence Hierarchy: Levels of Evidence

Level 1: Clinical Practice Guidelines based on evidence drawn from a comprehensive review and rating of available research studies and systematic reviews.

Level 2: Systematic reviews including integrated literature reviews and meta-analysis of experimental research studies.

Level 3: Single experimentally designed research studies.

Level 4: Systematic reviews including integrated literature reviews, meta-analysis, and metasynthesis of non-experimental/qualitative research studies.

Level 5: Single non-experimental or qualitative research studies.

Level 6: Non-research driven expert opinion or committee reports.

Adapted from Guyatt and Rennie (2002); Melnyk and Fineout-Overholt (2011); Polit and Beck (2008)

Resource and Subject Matter

The **evidence hierarchy** gives us a way to organize and rank any evidence that we have discovered from strongest to weakest. In this particular hierarchy, Level 1 is considered the strongest level of evidence and Level 6 is considered the weakest level of evidence. It is important to note, however, that the quality of evidence within a category may vary. Thus we need to evaluate the quality of the evidence as well as the level of evidence. For example in Level 1, clinical practice guidelines could be formulated by a national panel of experts using the best evidence available from all relevant research studies and SRRs. This would yield very high quality Level 1 evidence. On the other hand, if a clinical practice guideline was produced using sparse research evidence, or had not been subject to a rigorous review by experts, the resulting quality of the evidence would be suspect and might not offer the best support for practice.

The same is true of Level 2 or Level 4 systematic reviews. If the review uses a number of well-designed research studies and a well-formulated systematic approach to evaluating the studies, then the evidence produced is high quality. If few studies are available or if several of the studies are flawed, then the evidence produced may be of diminished quality. Level 3 and 5 refer to single research studies. Individual studies need to be well-designed and produce definitive results to be considered high quality evidence. Studies that have design problems, extremely small samples, or indeterminate or non-significant results are not very useful in providing supportive evidence.

Consider This . . .

How can an evidence hierarchy help you to determine which evidence is the best evidence?

There will always be clinical problems or questions where there is little research evidence available to guide your practice. When this occurs, it signals a need for research in that area. In the meantime, you will need to rely on clinical expertise, clinical experience, and evidence produced by the institution in which you work, such as policies, procedures, and data collected from quality improvement and risk assessments. This type of evidence is the lowest and weakest level of evidence (Level 6).

Let's examine a study that created havoc when picked up in the popular media. Check out *Research in the News* below.

Research in the News

Study: Autism Fraud

EDITORIAL NYTIMES.COM,
January 12, 2011

The report that first triggered scares that a vaccine to prevent measles, mumps and rubella might cause autism in children has received another devastating blow to its credibility. The British Medical Journal has declared that the research was not simply bad science, as has been known for years, but a deliberate fraud.

The study, led by Dr. Andrew Wakefield, was published in The Lancet in 1998. It was based on just 12 children with supposedly autism like disorders and purported to find a link between the vaccine, the gastrointestinal problems found in many autistic children, and autism.

While parents around the world were understandably alarmed, many scientists rejected the claims, including, eventually, 10 of Dr. Wakefield's co-authors. A high-level British medical group, after an exhaustive fitness-to-practice hearing, found Dr. Wakefield guilty of dishonesty and misconduct. The Lancet retracted the article in part, it said, because the authors had made false claims about how the study was conducted.

Now the British Medical Journal has taken the extraordinary step of publishing a lengthy report by Brian Deer, the British investigative journalist who first brought the paper's flaws to light—and has put its own reputation on the line by endorsing his findings.

After seven years of studying medical records and interviewing parents and doctors, Mr. Deer concluded that the medical histories of all 12 children had been misrepresented to make the vaccine look culpable. Time lines, for example, were fudged to make it seem as though *autism-like symptoms developed shortly after vaccination, while in some cases problems developed before vaccination and in others months after vaccination.*

Dr. Wakefield has accused Mr. Deer of being a hit man. But the medical journal compared the claims with evidence compiled in the voluminous transcript of official hearings and declared that flaws in the paper were not honest mistakes but rather an "elaborate fraud."

Some parents still consider Dr. Wakefield a hero, and others have moved on to other theories, equally unsupported by scientific evidence, as to how vaccines might cause autism.

They need to recognize that failure to vaccinate their children leaves them truly vulnerable to diseases that can cause enormous harm.

Here is a report that declares a 1998 research study on the connection between vaccines and autism to be fraudulent. This 1998 study and the reports of the results in the popular press aroused widespread fears and caused many parents to choose not to vaccinate their children.

Many subsequent research studies discounted the 1998 study but received little notice and widespread concerns about vaccines persisted.

Scan the original research study:

Wakefield, A.J. et al. 1998. Ileal-lymphoid-nodular hyperplasia, non-specific colitis, and pervasive developmental disorder in children. *The Lancet, 351*(9103): 637–641.

How do you suppose a non-experimental research study involving only 12 participants had such a huge impact on the general public in the first place? Would you have graded this study as a good piece of evidence?

What role might the popular press have played in spreading the initial fears? Were your opinions on vaccines influenced by the reports on the study?

The article was retracted by *The Lancet* (the journal which published the original article) in February 2010. The public controversy continued.

Do you think that coverage of the fraud by the popular press such as the article on the left can help increase vaccine rates among children? Did it affect your viewpoint?

What responsibility do you think the press has in reporting on scientific research studies?

Process for Using Evidence in Practice

In the same way that the nursing process guides practice and the research process guides the conduct of research studies, a process also helps to integrate evidence into nursing practice. This process, adapted from Melnyk and Fineout-Overholt (2011), and introduced in Chapter 1 of this text, has six steps:

1. problem identification
2. evidence collection
3. evidence appraisal
4. evidence integration and intervention implementation
5. outcome evaluation
6. outcome dissemination

IDENTIFYING CLINICAL PROBLEMS—FORM THE QUESTION. Problems arise from two major sources: either the clinician is presented with a problem which needs a solution in the course of clinical practice, or a problem is uncovered in the course of reading the literature or viewing a newly issued clinical guideline. In either case, the important thing is to determine whether the problem is significant enough to merit a change in the current practice. Evidence-based solutions can originate with the individual nurse who discovers a clinical problem in the course of everyday practice or from administration in an organization searching for a solution to an institution-wide problem.

Problems may be stated in a number of ways. Some are broad-based questions, such as "What is the best way to prevent deep vein thrombosis?" or "What is the best way to prevent asthma attacks?" Other questions may be more narrowly focused, such as "Are knee high TED hose as effective as thigh high TED hose in preventing deep vein thrombosis following surgery?" The first thing that you need to do is learn how to ask questions about your clinical practice in a way that is meaningful, searchable, and answerable. There are also a number of formats to guide the asking of a clinical question. We are going to use the **PICO(T)** approach presented by Melnyk and Fineout-Overholt (2011). They call for five parts to be identified when framing a clinical question: the **P**opulation, the **I**ntervention (or Interest), the **C**omparison intervention, the **O**utcome, and the **T**ime frame.

The "P" in PICO(T) stands for population, which denotes the characteristics of the patients or clients for whom the intervention is intended. For example, is the population

---

BOX 9-7 PICO(T)

	PICO(T) Format
P	population
I	intervention (interest)
C	comparison intervention
O	outcomes
T	time

children, teenagers, or adults? Is it male or female? Inpatients or outpatients? Do population members share a particular medical diagnosis? The "I" can stand for a particular intervention or a broader area of interest. For example, an intervention might be the use of gel-based handwashing products or the use of electronic thermometers. A question related to an area of interest can include a diagnosis or assessment, a prognosis, an etiology, or a meaning or process. Meaning and process questions are usually used when you want to provide insight into a particular phenomenon, to understand what the patient is going through, or to examine how culture influences patient care. Meaning questions usually make heavy use of qualitative research studies and metasyntheses. In this text, we focus on clinical interventions. The more specifically you define the intervention the more focused your search and answers will be.

The "C" in PICO(T) denotes a comparison, which can be an alternative intervention or the status quo. For example, you might ask about the effectiveness of gel-based handwashing products compared to soap and water, or the accuracy of electronic versus mercury-based thermometers. The "O" stands for outcomes or the consequences of the intervention. For instance, we want to determine the effectiveness (outcome) of two handwashing techniques or the accuracy (outcome) of two temperature measuring techniques in our two examples above. The "(T)" stands for time and specifies the time it takes for the intervention to achieve the outcome. The time frame is optional and not appropriate in all questions. Therefore we will represent it as "(T)". In the handwashing technique study the time frame might be after a 30 second wash.

If you need some assistance in wording a clinical question, try using the following template: In _____ (population), what is the effect of _____ (intervention) compared to _____ (comparison intervention) on _____ (outcome) within _____ (time frame). A PICO(T)-based question for our handwashing example might be: In *health care personnel working on a hospital orthopedic unit*, what is the effect of *using an alcohol-based hand gel* compared to *traditional handwashing techniques* on *the effectiveness of hand disinfection after a 30 second wash*? Our thermometer example can be stated without a time frame. For example, we might ask: In *adult patients on a general medical unit*, what is the effect of *using a head scan electronic thermometer compared to a glass mercury thermometer (gold standard)* on *the accuracy of temperature measurements*? The key to learning how to form good clinical questions is practice. Think about situations you have encountered in your clinical experiences. Identify a problem that you have observed in those experiences. Try using the template to formulate a question for that problem. Box 9-8 provides you with some more examples using the PICO(T) question format.

Consider This . . .

How does the PICO(T) approach help you focus on and define the clinical problem you want to address?

COLLECT THE EVIDENCE—SEARCHING THE LITERATURE. Once you have formulated a clinical question, the next step is to gather the evidence from the literature. Here is where the search skills you mastered in Chapter 2 come in handy. Your search needs to be approached systematically using the various databases available to you (see Chapter 2 and pages 199–200 in this chapter). If your question is focused and well-formulated it often

> ## BOX 9-8 Sample PICO(T) Questions
>
> **Question Template:**
> In _____ (population), what is the effect of _____ (intervention) compared to _____ (comparison intervention) on _____ (outcome) within _____ (time frame)?
>
> **Example 1:** In <u>children under age 5</u> (population), what is the effect of <u>using the FLACC observational pain assessment scale</u> (intervention) compared to <u>the FACES subjective pain scale</u> (comparison intervention) <u>on assessment of pain</u> (outcome)?
>
> **Example 2:** In <u>adult patients receiving chemotherapy</u> (population), what is the effect of <u>using oral cryotherapy in conjunction with oral hygiene</u> compared to <u>oral hygiene alone</u> (comparison intervention) <u>on preventing the development of oral mucositis</u> (outcome) <u>during course of chemotherapy</u> (time frame)?
>
> **Example 3:** In <u>adult patients undergoing hip surgery</u> (population), what is the effect of <u>using a no sting barrier film before taping the surgical site</u> compared to <u>no barrier film between the skin and tape</u> (comparison intervention) on <u>preventing skin blistering and breakdown</u> (outcome) <u>after surgery</u> (time frame)?

helps to look for summaries, systematic reviews, and clinical guidelines first. If you find ample evidence through reviews and/or clinical guidelines, you may not need to search for individual research studies to answer your question. So begin by checking out databases for systematic reviews such as the Cochrane and DARE databases and see if any IRRs, meta-analyses, or metasyntheses exist that address your question.

> ### Consider This . . .
>
> If you are having trouble with your evidence collection, be sure to review Chapter 2 for a systematic approach to the task.

Don't forget to search for CATs and information sheets. Then check out the National Guidelines Clearinghouse database and other applicable guideline databases to see if any clinical guidelines exist for your question. If there are no guidelines or systematic reviews, or if the ones you find were not published within the last 10 years (and thus are out of date), then you will need to proceed with a search for individual research articles that can provide evidence for your question. Select a comprehensive database such as *CINAHL* or MEDLINE. Remember to set up your search parameters. Your PICO(T) question should provide you with good direction in deciding on the parameters to use. The intervention, the comparison, and the outcome provides you with some key terms. The population helps you place limits on the search. Once you have searched all appropriate databases and collected all the relevant materials pertaining to your question, you are ready to move to Step 3.

APPRAISING THE EVIDENCE. Once you have collected the evidence, you need some way to organize it and determine what will be useful in answering your particular question. This can seem like an overwhelming task, particularly if you have found a great deal of evidence. You need a strategy for examining the various articles and reports that you have found. Remember that you are looking for the best possible evidence. This means that you are looking for research studies, systematic reviews of research studies, or clinical guidelines based on research studies as your first line of evidence.

> **Consider This . . .**
>
> Your first step in appraising the evidence might be to separate the collected evidence into four piles: 1) clinical guidelines, 2) systematic reviews, 3) individual research studies, and 4) non-research materials.

Start with the clinical guidelines and examine the following issues: summary, credibility, and applicability. This will allow you to determine who developed the guidelines, whether they are current, and whether they are based on research evidence. It also allows you to decide whether the guidelines would fit into your institution and whether they could be used in your clinical practice. The worksheet in Box 9-9 will help you address

---

BOX 9-9 Worksheet for Clinical Guidelines Appraisal

Citation: (Use the citation format used by your institution)

Summary:

List issues addressed by the guideline. _____

List clinical outcomes the guideline is attempting to achieve. _____

List population (audience) the guideline was intended for. _____

List the date that the guidelines were formulated or revised. _____

List the groups that produced the guidelines. _____

	Yes	No
Credibility:		
Did the people on the development panel possess the necessary expertise?	_____	_____
Was a systematic search for research evidence conducted?	_____	_____
Are the criteria for evidence selected stated?	_____	_____
Are the sources of the research evidence cited?	_____	_____
Are the guidelines current?	_____	_____
Have the guidelines been clinically tested?	_____	_____
Is the decision making process clearly spelled out?	_____	_____
Are the intended outcomes of implementing the guideline clearly stated?	_____	_____
Applicability:		
Does the guideline or part of the guideline specifically address the question that you asked?	_____	_____
Would the guidelines fit in your clinical setting?	_____	_____
Are the guidelines specific enough to guide your care?	_____	_____

continued. . .

	Yes	No
continued. . .		
Is the population addressed in the guideline compatible with the population in your setting?	_____	_____
Are patient risks clearly addressed?	_____	_____
Are there tools available to measure whether outcomes are met?	_____	_____
What changes would you have to make to adapt the guidelines?	_____	
Who would be affected by adaptation of the guidelines?	_____	

Evidence Level _____   **Evidence Quality** _____

each of these issues. You will note that the worksheet also makes space for you to rate the evidence. The evidence level comes from the evidence hierarchy in Box 9-6, and in the case of clinical guidelines, the evidence will be Level 1. A space for rating overall evidence quality is also available. You may rate the evidence quality as high (definitely credible and applicable), medium (credible but some applicability issues), or low (issues with credibility and/or applicability).

Next tackle the pile of systematic reviews. We will examine the same basic issues of summary, credibility, and applicability. Note that it is important to determine whether the review is addressing the same or similar interventions to the ones that you have identified in your question. You also need to know the number and type of studies used in the review and determine whether the conclusions would support the development of a protocol for the intervention that you have identified. Box 9-10 will provide you with a handy worksheet. Be sure to remember that systematic reviews are either Level 2 or Level 4 evidence depending on the types of research studies reviewed. Again, rate the quality of the review as high (definitely credible and applicable), medium (credible but some applicability issues), or low (issues with credibility and/or applicability). Hint: Any review that is produced by the Cochrane library has been subjected to the most rigorous of standards and the review is constantly being updated.

Now tackle the individual studies that you located. We will again look at the issues of summary, credibility, and applicability. The worksheet in Box 9-11 will help you with this task. Your level of evidence will depend on the study design. An experimental study produces Level 3 evidence. Non-experimental and qualitative studies produce Level 5 evidence. Evidence quality is high if the study is a well-developed peer reviewed study that uses your intervention and your population. A medium rating means that there may be minor flaws in the study or a less-than-adequate fit between the intervention or the population. A low rating would indicate issues with the study methods or with applicability to your question.

Now look at the remaining materials and ask yourself if there is anything useful to be gleaned about your problem. Cite the source and a brief summary of key points on a worksheet. Remember from the hierarchy that this evidence from non-research sources has an evidence level of six.

Once you have completed your appraisal of the various types of evidence, you need to appraise the nature of the intervention. An intervention which affects patient safety or involves a large investment of time and resources requires stronger support than one that

BOX 9-10 Worksheet for Systematic Review Appraisal

Citation: (Use the citation format used by your institution)

Summary:

List topic addressed by the systematic review. _____

List type of systematic review done (IRR, meta-analysis,
    metasynthesis). _____

List number of studies included in review. _____

List the dates covered in the search. _____

Describe the types of studies reviewed (experimental, non-experimental,
    qualitative). _____

List population targeted by the review. _____

Summarize the conclusions made by the review. _____

Describe any recommendations made by the review. _____

	Yes	No
Credibility:		
Was topic clearly defined?	____	____
Were search strategies of the literature described? (e.g., databases used, search terms used, limits of search)?	____	____
Are the criteria stated for the studies included or excluded?	____	____
Were studies used current? (within last 10 years)	____	____
Were conclusions of the review well supported by the studies used?	____	____
Applicability:		
Does the review specifically address the question that you asked?	____	____
Is the population addressed in the review compatible with the population in your setting?	____	____
Are the treatments or interventions similar to your intervention?	____	____
Could you devise a protocol for implementation using these conclusions?	____	____
Would incorporating the conclusions into a protocol create any barriers in implementation? (personnel, time, costs)	____	____

Evidence Level _____ **Evidence Quality** _____

entails no patient risk and requires little effort to implement. You must also appraise the collection of evidence as a whole to determine whether you have enough evidence and whether it is strong enough to support your intervention. You need to determine whether the findings in your evidence will transfer to your particular situation. You also need to determine what factors are involved in implementing a protocol for the intervention. How feasible is it to change to this intervention? Ultimately you need to make a decision about adopting or rejecting the intervention. Box 9-12 contains a worksheet to help you with these decisions.

BOX 9-11 Worksheet for Individual Research Study Appraisal

Citation: (Use the citation format used by your institution)

Summary:

List the purpose of the study (research questions, hypotheses, aims, or objectives). _____

Identify the variables/phenomena. _____

Identify the population and the sample. _____

Identify the study design (experimental, non-experimental, or qualitative). _____

Describe any intervention or treatment. _____

Identify sample number and sampling technique. _____

Identify the instruments used. _____

Identify data analysis procedures (statistics or theme derivation process). _____

Describe the sample characteristics. _____

Summarize the results. _____

	Yes	No
Credibility:		
Was the article peer reviewed?	___	___
Was the research problem clearly identified?	___	___
Were the research questions answered?	___	___
Were the instruments reliable and valid?	___	___
Was the sample large enough to find a significant outcome?	___	___
If statistics were used, were the findings significant?	___	___
Were the limitations of the study identified?	___	___
Applicability:		
Does this study examine your intervention or comparison intervention of interest?	___	___
Does this study use a sample similar to your population of interest?	___	___
Do the results help support your intervention of interest?	___	___

Evidence Level _____   **Evidence Quality** _____

Consider This . . .

What factors must be considered before you can decide whether to use an intervention?

INTEGRATE THE EVIDENCE AND IMPLEMENT THE INTERVENTION. Once you have decided to adopt the intervention, it must be integrated into practice. Integrating the evidence makes use of the last two features of the definition for evidence-based practice that we

BOX 9-12 Worksheet for Body of Evidence Appraisal

	Yes	No
Intervention:		
Is patient safety a factor in implementing the intervention?	_____	_____
Is patient satisfaction a factor?	_____	_____
What costs are associated with implementing the intervention?	_____	
What personnel resources are needed to implement the intervention?	_____	
Quality of Evidence:		
How many Level 1 through 3 studies support the intervention?	_____	
How many Level 4 and 5 studies support the intervention?	_____	
What was the overall quality of the evidence? (high, medium, low)	_____	
Transferability:		
Are the populations in a majority of studies similar with the population at your institution?	_____	_____
Is your institution similar to the study settings?	_____	_____
How many participants would be affected by the intervention?	_____	
Feasibility:		
Is there institutional support for the intervention?	_____	_____
Does staff have the skills to implement the intervention?	_____	_____
Does the intervention add to staff workload?	_____	_____
What are possible barriers and facilitators to implementing this intervention?	_____	

Adop _____ **Consider a Pilot Project** _____ **Do Not Adopt** _____

explored at the beginning of this chapter: fitting individual patient needs and preferences. Communication and involvement of the patient in care-giving decisions is important. Any qualitative research that you reviewed in your evidence appraisal may give you keys to how the patient might feel about a particular intervention. Finally, clinical expertise is key in integrating decisions into a specified care setting. The clinician's assessment of the situation, the needs of the patient, the availability of resources, and the skills required to implement the intervention will help determine the success of the intervention. If the intervention is a simple one, it may be carried out relatively easily.

For example, suppose your unit uses both knee high and thigh high TED hose and the choice of which to use rests with the nurse. You know that many patients will wear the knee high stockings, but will often take the thigh high stockings off or refuse to wear them because they are too hot and uncomfortable. You don't know whether the patients receive the same benefit from knee high stockings. You ask the PICOT question: In adult general medical patients (P), what is the effect of knee high TED stockings (I) compared to thigh high TED stocking (C) on improving circulation and the prevention of deep venous thromboses (DVTs) (O) during a hospital stay (T)? You find a number of Level 2 and Level 3 studies that show knee high stockings are as effective as the thigh high stockings at improving circulation and preventing DVTs. You now feel secure in offering patients a choice of stocking. As you implement the choice, you decide to keep track of the choices and the use of the stockings.

Interventions that require staff training, equipment, and/or supplies usually require a protocol so that everyone in the institution is on the same page. Protocols are often developed by a committee and are tailored for the particular institution and patient population affected. Protocols list the purpose of the protocol, the rational for the protocol, the expected clinical outcomes, the steps for implementation of the intervention, and a reference list of the supporting research.

> **Consider This . . .**
>
> What sort of roadblocks might there be when moving from identifying an intervention to adopting it?

EVALUATE THE OUTCOMES. Step 5 in evidence-based practice is to evaluate the effectiveness of the implementation of intervention. The intended outcome that was stated in your PICO(T) question from Step 1 serves as a guideline for evaluation. If the change was a simple one, the evaluation may be fairly informal. You, as an individual clinician, might chart whether the desired outcome was reached. If the implementation of the intervention was more complex and occurred by use of a protocol, then protocol outcomes serve as the guiding direction for the evaluation. Our example would call for a more formal evaluation. Evaluation needs to take into account the overall effectiveness of the intervention from a unit or institutional perspective as viewed by certain predetermined benchmarks and using prescribed measurement tools. Costs and benefits are also likely to be evaluated.

DISSEMINATE THE OUTCOMES. The final step in the process is to share the results of the evidence-based change that was implemented and evaluated. In our example, if you discovered that patients on your unit wore knee highs more consistently and for longer periods of time, then you need to share these findings with colleagues. This begins by sharing the results with your own institution. You might present an inservice or use a podcast or hold a roundtable discussion. You also need to share your findings with other health care professionals. This can be done through poster or podium presentations at local, regional, or national professional conferences. The most effective and widespread way to get the message out is through publication in a professional journal.

We will be examining some specific examples of evidence-based interventions in Chapter 10. As a student or practicing nurse, you may find and support many of your nursing actions with research. Each time you back your practice decisions with research evidence, you are making a conscious effort to use the best evidence in making clinical decisions about the care that you render. This is a habit well worth developing and will serve you well throughout your nursing career.

SUMMARY

In this chapter, you have been introduced to a number of resources, an evidence hierarchy, and an evidence-based practice process involving five steps and several question formulation examples and appraisal worksheets. Here is a summary of the key points in this chapter.

- **Evidence-based practice** makes use of research-based materials to provide a systematic approach to investigate and provide solutions to clinical problems.

Research utilization, which can be classified as conceptual, instrumental, or persuasive, starts with research findings and moves to seeking practical applications. EBP starts with the identification of a clinical problem and seeks research-based evidence to support decision-making. *(Objective 1)*

• Many **evidence-based (EB) models** exist that provide a specific process to guide the EBP process and bring a change in clinical practice. Key models are the IOWA, Stetler, ACE Star, and Rosswurm/Larrabee. *(Objective 2)*

• Evidence can be drawn from individual research studies, **systematic reviews**, **clinical practice guidelines**, synopses of systematic reviews, **critically appraised topics (CATs)**, and best practice information sheets. Common types of systematic reviews include **integrative research reviews (IRR), systematic research reviews (SRR), meta-analyses**, and **metasyntheses**. *(Objective 3)*

• Evidence is rated using an **evidence hierarchy** to determine the level (from weakest—Level 6 to strongest—Level 1) and quality (from high to low) of the available evidence. *(Objective 4)*

• A five-step process for using evidence in practice provides structure for identifying a clinical problem, collecting evidence, appraising evidence, implementing an intervention, and evaluating outcomes. *(Objective 5)*

• **PICO(T)** provides a structured approach for identifying a clinical problem and identifies the target **P**opulation, the **I**ntervention/Interest, the **C**omparison intervention, **O**utcomes, and **T**ime. *(Objective 6)*

• Once the problem is identified, evidence must be collected and appraised using specified appraisal criteria in order to find a specific intervention and then to determine whether to adopt that intervention. If a decision is made to adopt an intervention, the evidence must be integrated and the intervention implemented in practice. Once a change in clinical practice occurs, outcomes must evaluated to determine whether the targeted intervention was effective and cost-effective. Results of a successful outcome need to be shared with professional colleagues. *(Objective 7)*

Now it is time for you to see whether you can apply what you have learned.

STUDENT ACTIVITIES

1. Locate the following integrative review: Vanderbloom, T. 2007. Does music reduce anxiety during invasive procedures with procedural sedation? An integrative research review. *Journal of Radiology Nursing, 26*(1): 15–22. What does this review tell you about whether the use of music can reduce anxiety during invasive procedures?

2. Pull up the following link www.rnao.org/Storage/50/4488_Oral_Health-Jan9.09-web.pdf to the clinical practice guideline on oral hygiene. Look at the summary of the guideline on pages 10–11. How might you use these guidelines in the clinical area?

3. As you look at the practice guidelines on oral hygiene on pages 10–11 of the link, you notice that the evidence is marked as level III or level IV. What does that mean? (Hint: look at page 12 of the report.)

4. Do a search for "Critically appraised topics in Nursing" using your internet search engine. What did you find out about CATs? How might you use CATs?

5. Now locate the following article: Steel, S. 2005. Using critically appraised topics to inform nursing practice in DVT prevention using graduated compression stockings. *Journal of Orthopaedic Nursing, 9*(4): 211–217. What did you learn about using CATs from this article? How would this CAT be useful in your clinical practice?

Pearson Nursing Student Resources

Find additional review materials at

www.nursing.pearsonhighered.com

Prepare for success with additional NCLEX®-style practice questions, interactive assignments and activities, web links, animations and videos, and more!

REFERENCES

Estabrooks, C.A. 1999. The conceptual structure of research utilization. *Research in Nursing and Health, 22*(3): 203.

Guyatt, G. and D. Rennie. 2002. *User's guides to medical literature.* American Medical Association: AMA Press.

Ingersoll, G. 2000. Evidence-based nursing: What it is and what it isn't. *Nursing Outlook, 48*(4): 151–152.

Melnyk, B. and E. Fineout-Overholt. 2011. *Evidence-based practice in nursing and healthcare.* New York, NY: Lippincott Williams & Wilkins.

Polit, D.F. and C.T. Beck. 2008. *Nursing research, generating and assessing evidence for nursing practice.* New York, NY: Lippincott Williams & Wilkins.

Rosswurm, M.A. and J. Larrabee. 1999. A model for change to evidence-based practice. *Image: Journal of Nursing Scholarship, 31*(4): 317–322.

Steel, S. 2005. Using critically appraised topics to inform nursing practice in DVT prevention using graduated compression stockings. *Journal of Orthopaedic Nursing, 9(4):* 211–217.

Stetler, C.B. 2001. Updating the Stetler model of research utilization to facilitate evidence-based practice. *Nursing Outlook, 49:* 272–278.

Stetler, C.B. and G. Marram. 1976. Evaluating research findings for applicability in practice. *Nursing Outlook, 24:* 559–563.

Stevens, K.R. 2004. ACE Star Model of EBP: Knowledge Transformation. Academic Center for Evidence-based Practice. www.acestar.uthscsa.edu.

Titler, M.G., C. Klieber, V. Steelman, C. Goode, B. Rakel, J. Barry-Walker, S. Small, and K. Buckwalter. 1994. Infusing research into practice to promote quality care. *Nursing Research , 43*(5): 307–313.

Titler, M.G., C. Klieber, V. Steelman, B. Rakel, G. Budreau, L. Everett, K. Buckwalter, T. Tripp-Reimer, and C. Goode. 2001. The Iowa Model of evidence based practice to promote quality care. *Critical Care Nursing Clinics of North America, 13:* 497–509.

Vanderbloom, T. 2007. Does music reduce anxiety during invasive procedures with procedural sedation? An integrative research review. *Journal of Radiology Nursing, 26*(1): 15–22.

Whittemore, R. 2005. Combining evidence in Nursing research: Methods and implications. *Nursing Research, 54*(1): 56–62.

Yick, A. 2008. A metasynthesis of qualitative findings on the role of spirituality and religiosity among culturally diverse domestic violence survivors. *Qualitative Health Research, 18*(9): 1289–1306.

Zhou, H., P. Roberts, and L. Horgan. 2008. Association between self-report pain ratings of child and parent, child and nurse and parent and nurse dyads: meta-analysis. *Journal of Advanced Nursing, 63*(4): 334–342.

Putting Research Evidence into Practice

CHAPTER OUTLINE

CHAPTER OBJECTIVES

1. Apply the EBP model to identifying a clinical problem.
2. Apply the EBP model to the process of collecting evidence.
3. Apply the EBP model to evidence appraisal.
4. Apply the EBP model to integrating evidence in order to implement an intervention.
5. Apply the EBP model to evaluating the outcome of the intervention.
6. Apply the EBP model to plan a strategy for disseminating outcomes.

KEY TERMS

Clinical problem (**p. 217**)   Evidence integration (**p. 225**)

Evidence appraisal (**p. 222**)   Outcome evaluation (**p. 234**)

ABSTRACT

Evidence-based practice is a process guided by a systematic, step-by-step approach to integrating research findings into practice. In Chapter 9 you learned about the six key steps: (1) problem identification, (2) evidence collection, (3) evidence appraisal, (4) evidence integration and intervention implementation, (5) outcome evaluation, and (6) outcome dissemination. This chapter applies each of those steps to a running example of developing a hand hygiene protocol.

In Chapter 9 you were introduced to models of evidence-based practice (EBP). This chapter is all about applying the EBP process. Here, we will actually select a model and apply the process to a common nursing problem: infection control. This chapter will be divided according to the six steps of the EBP process, as follows: (1) identifying the problem, (2) collecting the evidence, (3) appraising the evidence, (4) integrating the evidence and implementing the intervention, (5) evaluating the outcome, and (6) disseminating the outcomes. We will systematically work through these steps, following a team of nurses as they apply them to a clinical problem.

Step 1: Identify the Clinical Problems—Form the Question

In patient care situations, infection control is a critical issue. Nosocomial (hospital-acquired) infections increase morbidity and mortality, resulting in increased expense and extended lengths of stays. Moreover, some hospital-acquired infections are no longer reimbursed by Medicare and Medicaid. Consequently, all patient care providers want to find ways of preventing infections. A potential change is on the horizon at 6 North, Hope Hospital's orthopedic unit, where a high percentage of patients undergo hip, knee, and shoulder replacements: hand hygiene. While all care providers are taught about regular handwashing, there is a possibility that alcohol gels may be made available for hand cleaning on entry to patient rooms. Let's face it, washing and drying hands correctly takes time. What if you could substitute an alcohol gel that would be much more convenient and time-saving? While 6 North's nurses feel that using an alcohol gel might be quicker and easier than handwashing, they express concern that alcohol gels may be less effective in preventing infection.

Before the nurses realize it, they have identified a **clinical problem** (a patient care situation encountered in nursing practice that requires a solution) and started the process of gathering evidence to determine best clinical practice.

Consider This . . .

Based on your experiences in nursing to date, what kind of clinical problems can you identify that would be good to investigate? How might you get the process started?

Think back to the prior chapter. The first steps in evidence-based practice (EBP) are identifying the problem and forming the question. Recall that the PICO(T) format—with P standing for the patient population, I for intervention or interest, C for comparison intervention, O for outcomes, and (T) for time—can provide a template for formulating a clinical question. So what would a question look like for the problem the nurses identified?

P: The patient *population* is adult, orthopedic patients undergoing hip, knee, and shoulder replacements.

I: The proposed *intervention* is requiring health care professionals to use alcohol hand gel on entering patient rooms.

C: The *comparison* is between health care professionals using soap and water handwashing versus alcohol gels on entering the patient room.

O: The *outcome* is the rate of unit infections.

(T): The *time* is unspecified.

So, how might the nurses phrase their clinical question? *In adult orthopedic patients who are undergoing joint replacements, what is the effect of health care providers using alcohol hand gel when entering patient rooms compared with traditional soap and water handwashing on unit infection rates?*

Are all of the pieces here? Use Figure 10-1 to make sure.

Patient	Intervention	Comparison	Outcome
Adult orthopedic patients undergoing joint replacements	Health care providers using alcohol hand gel	Traditional soap and water handwashing	Unit infection rates

■ **FIGURE 10-1** Problem Statement Components

Step 2: Collect the Evidence by Searching the Literature

Recall that Chapter 2 of this text discussed searching for research evidence. This chapter will employ those techniques. So, it may be a good time to brush up on the search methods, which will be used in the following example. The steps of literature review introduced in

Chapter 2 will guide this section. These include: (1) define and refine the topic, (2) select appropriate resources, (3) choose appropriate databases, (4) define search parameters and run search, (5) examine search results, and (6) collect resources from search.

Define and Refine Topic

To begin a search one must know enough about the topic and associated key concepts in order to appropriately narrow the search parameters. Nurses on the Orthopedic Unit began their discussion by identifying key concepts associated with their problem. They made a chart like Table 10-1 to summarize the results of their discussion.

▶ Table 10-1 Concepts and Key Words for Hand Hygiene, Infection, and Orthopedic Patients	
Subject Area	**Hand Hygiene**
Key concepts & sub-concepts	Infection prevention Hand hygiene Handwashing Alcohol gels
Population	Adult orthopedic patients undergoing joint replacements
Narrow focus	Effectiveness of an intervention: soap and water handwashing versus quick drying alcohol hand gels
Key concepts/Key words	Infection prevention Joint replacement patients Hand hygiene
Final refined topic	Influence of using handwashing versus alcohol gels on unit infection rates

Select Appropriate Resources

Sometimes, a good way to start a search of a new topic is to check a general source: try a quick look using Google or examine nursing texts regarding handwashing or infection control. Remember, this is just a way to get the search started, but there are other places to go in order to obtain the evidence on which to base a change in practice. A Google check reveals 1,890,000 hits for hand hygiene! That is fairly overwhelming. However, there is a wonderful piece of information in the first citation—a link to the Centers for Disease Control and Prevention (CDC) Hand Hygiene Guidelines written in 2002 (Boyce and Pittet 2002). This document is an important piece of information as the nurses begin to build their evidence.

Choose Appropriate Databases

As mentioned in Chapter 2, two of the most commonly used databases for nursing research are the Cumulative Index to Nursing and Allied Health Literature (*CINAHL*) and Medical Literature Online (MEDLINE). Other useful sources may be the Cochrane Database of Systematic Reviews and any clinical guidelines that are available.

Define Parameters and Run Search

The two steps of defining search parameters and running a search go hand in hand. When defining parameters, key words are selected to use as search terms. Defining parameters and running the search allows discovery of additional information that guides decision making. Once the initial search is completed, the nurses might try a new set of parameters and continue narrowing the search field, or they might decide to remove some of the limits previously set.

The nurses begin by entering one of the key terms: hand hygiene. In *CINAHL*, this term yielded 812 hits—not a particularly large number for a topic that should be fairly broad (remember, there were over a million hits in Google). While *hand hygiene* is an encompassing term that incorporates the concept of both handwashing and alcohol gel use, the nurses begin to wonder if by using it they are missing articles that simply use the term *handwashing* rather than *hand hygiene. Hand hygiene* is a term that has appeared in the literature more recently (Bjerke 2004; Boyce and Pittet 2002). Remember the concept of Boolean operators that you learned about in Chapter 2? These are words such as AND or OR that link together key terms that can be used in a search. So, what happens to the search if the nurses add a Boolean operator of OR to search for Hand Hygiene OR Handwashing? The search results are somewhat different with 3,366 articles related to hand hygiene or handwashing (and 3,867 hits in MEDLINE). This initial number is more in line with what the nurses anticipated; they're on the right path. Table 10-2 shows the citation count as the nurses proceed with the search process.

▶ Table 10-2   Search Strategy for Hand Hygiene/Handwashing Citations

Key Words/Limits	CINAHL Hits	MEDLINE Hits
Hand hygiene OR Handwashing	3,366	3,867
Gels (*CINAHL*)	53	
Handwashing method (MEDLINE MeSH Heading)		551
Infection Control	17	67
Research	7	

Consider This . . .

The search for resources has begun. How do you know when it is time to stop narrowing the search and begin to acquire the discovered resources?

Since it is not productive to examine this number of references, the nurses need to refine their search further. In *CINAHL*, one of the ways to limit a search is to use the Major Subject Headings area found on the search screen. A Major Subject Heading regarding handwashing is Gels, one of the key concepts discussed in this project. When the term *gels* is introduced, the number of relevant articles drops to fifty-three, and that number is further reduced to seventeen when the term *Infection Control* is entered (also one of the major topic headings that can be selected). Rather than Major Subject Headings, MEDLINE uses the term *MeSH* or *Medical Subject Heading* which is a directory that indexes the database of articles. MeSH headings allow a choice of Handwashing Method—rather than gels specifically. With this restriction, the number of MEDLINE citations is reduced to 551. Adding another MeSH heading of Infection Control Methods yields 67 potential articles in English. Now the nurses face a choice: research is not a MeSH heading in MEDLINE, yet many articles regarding handwashing and infection control are found in infection control journals, so they don't want to limit their search to nursing journals. At this point, they decide to end the search and sort through the possible alternatives.

Consider This . . .

The nurses have found a number of promising resources. Should they stop now? Why or why not?

One other resource to check out to ensure that no systematic literature reviews are missed is the Cochrane Database of Systematic Reviews. This yielded one additional systematic literature review on interventions to improve hand hygiene compliance in patient care (Gould, Chudleigh, Moralejo, and Drey 2007). The nurses added this review to their other citations.

Examine Search Results

It is time to examine the type of articles found in the search. Because evidence levels consist of research findings as well as research reviews and clinical guidelines, the nurses made the decision to examine the articles with citations they found when they added the search term infection control, including seventeen citations in *CINAHL* and sixty-seven citations in MEDLINE. While titles on the search list can give a sense of the contents of an article, reading the abstract is really the best way to determine how potentially useful the article might be. In order to save the searches, the nurses used temporary folders so they could access the searches later, when they had more time to read the articles or if further questions about the searches arose.

First, they considered the seventeen articles from the *CINAHL* search. One surprise was that a study on alcohol gels was actually conducted on an orthopedic unit. Rarely is an article so specific to the problem at hand. Additionally, there were both research and non-research materials that were relevant.

Consider This . . .

Stop and think! What criteria should be used to determine if an article should be reviewed or not? What can you do to get more information about the article? When you formulate your response to this question, move ahead.

Next, the nurses prioritized the articles requiring follow-up evaluation to determine their usefulness to the project. An important part of determining if a citation might be useful is to read the title and, most importantly, examine the abstract for the specifics. Box 10-1 contains some of the article titles as well as the categories used by the nurses to sort the articles based on the potential usefulness of the article. Remember, just because a citation made it through the search process does not necessarily mean that it is relevant to the proposed project—for instance, "Bedside Tipple" is clearly not about the right kind of alcohol!

A review of the seventeen titles left the nurses with 7 articles that they are sure they want to check and at least four others that may warrant further examination. Several of the "to keep" articles are research-based and deal with infection control in acute care settings (although one examines community settings). In the "maybe" list, some of the articles

---

BOX 10-1 Search Titles and Decisions Made from Hand Hygiene Search

Titles of Citations to Keep
- Effectiveness of hand hygiene procedures in reducing risks of infection in home and community settings, including handwashing and alcohol-based hand sanitizers
- Reduction in nosocomial transmission of drug-resistant bacteria after introduction of an alcohol-based hand rub
- Introduction of a waterless hand gel was associated with a reduced rate of ventilator-associated pneumonia in a surgical intensive care unit
- Comparative in vitro and in vivo study of nine alcohol-based hand rubs
- Differences in hand hygiene behavior related to the contamination risk of health care activities in different groups of health care workers
- Alcohol-based hand rub: Evaluation of technique and microbiological efficacy with international infection control professionals
- Use of alcohol hand sanitizer as an infection control strategy in an acute care facility

Titles Warranting Further Investigation
- Going dotty: A practical guide for installing new hand hygiene products
- Study links alcohol gel to fewer infections: But rubs should not be used in some outbreaks
- Limited efficacy of alcohol-based hand gels (letter)
- Alcohol-based hand gels and hand hygiene in hospitals (letter)

Titles of Citations to Eliminate
- Bedside Tipple
- Conducting a campaign to improve hand hygiene in non-acute health care
- Fire chiefs back alcohol hand rubs in hospitals: May lead to national code changes
- Fire and alcohol: Hand-hygiene plans getting hosed down by safety officials
- JCAHO addresses issue of fire, alcohol rubs: Install containers inside rooms, not halls

deal with the pragmatics of setting up an alcohol gel system while others deal with related topics of alcohol gel use for food workers or reflect some ongoing arguments between groups advocating for or against alcohol gel use. The nurses eliminated some citations even though they discussed alcohol gel use because they dealt with more peripherally related issues such as fire hazard considerations, a matter that has already been resolved.

Next, the nurses reviewed the sixty-seven citations and abstracts from the MEDLINE search. Not surprisingly, many of the same articles found in *CINAHL* also turned up in the MEDLINE search. The nurses reviewed any articles unique to the MEDLINE search for possible inclusion. A number of citations were eliminated because they did not specifically deal with the use of alcohol gel (remember, the MeSH heading option was handwashing methods rather than gels exclusively). A particularly important find in this search was a systematic literature review gathering study findings on hand hygiene.

Collect Resources from Search

In order to store the data, the nurses decided to download full texts to a computer file, then review the articles and print only those that contained particularly relevant information to the topic of handwashing and alcohol gel use.

> **Consider This . . .**
>
> As you are beginning to discover, gathering and evaluating information for an evidence-based practice project has many steps. What kind of things could you do make the process more manageable?

Step 3: Appraise the Evidence

The next step is examining the evidence collected by conducting an **evidence appraisal**. In EBP an evidence appraisal is the process of systematically evaluating literature and guidelines found that are relevant to a selected nursing problem. Approximately 15 articles or clinical guidelines were gathered and organized into the following topic areas.

- Infection reduction
- Microbial properties of alcohol gel rubs
- Techniques for hand hygiene
- Education and adherence to hand hygiene protocols

Some of the publications addressed more than one topic area, particularly systematic literature reviews. After reviewing the articles, the nurses eliminated some of them because they were out of date. For example, an excellent review and clinical guideline published by the Association for Professionals in Infection Control (Larson 1995) was eliminated because it was published in 1995 and did not incorporate more recent research that modified clinical practices regarding handwashing and alcohol gel use. It became more apparent that recent articles were going to be especially important.

Level 1: Clinical Practice Guidelines

Recall from Chapter 9 that clinical guidelines are considered to be one of the strongest levels of clinical evidence. Box 10-2 shows an appraisal of the CDC hand hygiene guidelines using the worksheet introduced in Chapter 9.

BOX 10-2 Worksheet for Clinical Guidelines Appraisal: CDC Hand Hygiene Guidelines

Citation:
Boyce, J. and D. Pittet. 2002. Guideline for hand hygiene in health-care settings: Recommendations of the Healthcare Infection Control Practices Advisory Committee and the HICPAC/SHEA/APIC Hand Hygiene Task Force. *Morbidity and Mortality Weekly Report, 51*(No. RR-16): 1–45.

Summary:
List issues addressed by the guideline.

- Reviews data regarding hand hygiene in health care settings, particularly with regard to research since 1985, the date of the last CDC recommendations.
- Specific recommendations based on data review made for implementation in health care arenas.
- Recommendations for a research agenda in education and promotion, hand hygiene agents and hand care, and laboratory based and epidemiologic research.

List clinical outcomes the guideline is attempting to achieve.

- Reduced transmission of nosocomial infections through adherence to hand hygiene guidelines.
- Improved research data regarding hand hygiene.

List population (audience) the guideline was intended for.

- Heath Care Workers.

List the date that the guidelines were formulated or revised.

- 2002; These continue to serve as guidelines in 2011.

List the groups that produced the guidelines.

- Centers for Disease Control and Prevention (CDC).
- Healthcare Infections Control Practices Advisory Committee (HICPAC).
- Society for Healthcare Epidemiology of America (SHEA).
- Association for Professionals in Infection Control (APIC).
- Infectious Diseases Society of America (IDSA).

	Yes	No
Credibility:		
Did the people on the development panel possess the necessary expertise?	X	

The twenty-one professionals on the taskforce were physicians, nurses, or public health officials who all had a history in hand hygiene as demonstrated by multiple publications—both research-based and review articles. Additionally, each of the professionals were active members in infection control organizations and served as representatives of those organizations on the task force developing the guidelines.

| Was a systematic search for research evidence conducted? | X | |

While a specific strategy for literature review was not described, 423 articles in English as well as other languages were cited. Research studies

continued . . .

continued . . .
ranged from non-experimental to experimental designs. Each of the areas addressed by the report provided multiple research citations.

	Yes	No

Are the criteria for evidence selected stated?   _____   X
While the strengths and shortcomings of studies are reviewed, specific criteria for inclusion as evidence are not stated.

Are the sources of the research evidence cited?   X   _____
Citations present throughout—including attaching citations to each of the final recommendations. Final guidelines are categorized:

• IA category recommendations are strongly recommended for clinical implementation and well supported by prior research.
• IB recommendations are supported by some research.
• IC are required items because it is legally mandated.
• Category II are suggestions for implementation and based on theory or clinical/epidemiologic study.
• The final category is no recommendation due to unresolved practice issues secondary to insufficient evidence.

Are the guidelines current?   X   _____
These are most recent set of recommendations on hand hygiene for health care providers set forth by a national body.

Have the guidelines been clinically tested?   _____   X
Recommendations for research in the area of education, hand hygiene agents and care, and laboratory-based research and development are made. There is no evidence of specific clinical testing for these guidelines.

Is the decision-making process clearly spelled out?   _____   X

Are the intended outcomes of implementing the guideline clearly stated?   X   _____
Performance indicators include monitoring (a) protocol adherence, (b) volume of alcohol rub or detergent used, (c) adherence to policies for use of artificial nails, and (d) infection outbreaks.

Applicability:
Does the guideline or part of the guideline specifically address the question that you asked?   X   _____
Specific behavioral recommendations regarding hand hygiene in clinical settings are made. Special cases are also considered.

Would the guidelines fit in our clinical setting?   X   _____
Recommendations are feasible in the proposed clinical setting. They will require additional equipment to dispense alcohol gel products.

Are the guidelines specific enough to guide your care?   X   _____
Guidelines are explicit regarding clinical situations.

Is the population addressed in the guideline compatible with the population in your setting?   X   _____
Guidelines are fairly universal to health care in general—adult orthopedic patients undergoing joint replacement would fit under this umbrella.

	Yes	No
Are patient risks clearly addressed?	____	_X_

Addresses risks of contact dermatitis for health care providers. Does not specifically address patient risks—if they exist.

| Are there tools available to measure whether outcomes are met? | _X_ | ____ |

- Adherence: direct observation of hand hygiene episodes
- Agents: monitor volume of alcohol rub and/or handwashing detergent
- Infection rates—occurrence
- Microbial counts

There are other recommendations for research that would require instrument development.

What changes would you have to make to adapt the guidelines?

- In order to incorporate alcohol gels on the clinical unit, a decision would need to be made regarding product.
- Alcohol gel dispensers would need to be installed in each patient room since fire codes sometimes prohibit installing the dispensers in halls of patient care areas.
- Health care worker education would be needed regarding the new policy.

Who would be affected by adaptation of the guidelines?

- All health care workers
- Policy and procedure committee—to develop and place procedure into manual
- Maintenance
- Housekeeping

Evidence Level: Level 1   **Evidence Quality: High**

While the CDC guideline did not perfectly address each of the questions, it is a strong, well respected document whose recommendations are based on available clinical research. At this point, this guideline is virtually the gold standard in the health care industry. It will be a key document as the nurses make their proposal to switch to alcohol gel.

Consider This . . .

The clinical guideline is a Level 1 piece of evidence. Do the nurses need to continue reading other potential sources of evidence? Why or Why not?

Level 2: Systematic Literature Reviews

Systematic literature reviews offer a means of **evidence integration** on a particular topic. Evidence integration uses the clinical expertise of the care provider, their assessment of the situation, and potentially input of patients combined with the evidence obtained in order to make decisions about implementation of an evidence-based plan (Melnyk and Fineout-Overholt 2011). In this project, the Cochrane Database contained a systematic literature review regarding interventions to improve

BOX 10-3 Worksheet for Systematic Review of Hand Hygiene Practice Adherence

Citation:
Gould, D., J. Chudleigh, D. Moralejo, and N. Drey. 2007. Interventions to improve hand hygiene compliance in patient care. *Cochrane Database of Systematic Reviews*, Issue 2. Art. No.:10.1002/14651858.CD005186.pub2.

Summary:
List topic addressed by the systematic review.

• Adherence to hand hygiene practices and influence of adherence on infection rates.

List type of systematic review done (IRR, meta-analysis, metasynthesis)

• Metasynthesis

List number of studies included in review.

• Two studies were included in the review—45 studies were excluded for not meeting study inclusion criteria.

List the dates covered in the search.

• 1986 to 2005

Describe the types of studies reviewed (experimental, non experimental, qualitative).

• Experimental

List population targeted by the review.

• Health care workers

Summarize the conclusions made by the review.

• Limited conclusions were described due to the limited number of studies that qualified for inclusion.

Describe any recommendations made by the review.

• Authors suggest that studies of compliance with hand hygiene protocols with strong experimental designs are important and need to be undertaken. These studies should be behavioral in nature and include theoretical underpinnings for intervention—particularly considering social-cognitive models.

	Yes	No
Credibility:		
Was topic clearly defined?	X	

Very clearly defined: Examined short and long term success of hand hygiene compliance and ascertained if health care related infection rates could be decreased by sustained hand hygiene compliance.

	Yes	No
Were search strategies of the literature described? (e.g., databases used, search terms used, limits of search)?	X	

Explicitly identified—included use of the Cochrane registry, MEDLINE, PubMed, EMBASE, *CINAHL*, and the BNI—searched between 1980 (MEDLINE), 1990 (remaining databases except *CINAHL* which was searched from inception) through 2006. Terms and search strategies explicitly delineated.

	Yes	No
Are the criteria stated for the studies included and excluded?	X	
Clearly stated. For inclusion, studies needed to be randomized control trials, controlled clinical trials, controlled before-and-after studies, or uninterrupted time series analyses.		
Were studies used current? (within last 10 years)	X	
1986 was the earliest study considered for inclusion—actual studies selected were from 1997 (within the 10-year period at time of review) and 2002		
Were conclusions of the review well supported by the studies used?	X	
The authors concluded that sufficient evidence did not exist due to poorly designed studies with short follow-up periods.		

Applicability:

	Yes	No
Does the review specifically address the question that you asked?	X	
Review addresses a relevant question: findings do not support specific intervention.		
Review addresses one aspect of implementing an alcohol gel rub system: compliance of health care workers in using the system.		
Is the population addressed in the review compatible with the population in your setting?	X	
Health care workers		
Are the treatments or interventions similar to your intervention?	X	
Authors recommended that intervention should include education and extended follow-up to check for sustained hand hygiene practices.		
Could you devise a protocol for implementation using these conclusions?	X	
Suggestions are given for potential practices— but applicability based on research is limited.		
Would incorporation of the conclusions into a protocol create any barriers in implementation? (personnel, time, costs)		X
Outcomes were inconclusive—recommendations regarding research may be useful.		

Evidence Level: Level 2   **Evidence Quality: Low**

hand hygiene compliance in patient care. Box 10-3 presents a worksheet for a sestematic review. This review is relevant to the nurses' project because selecting the right gel is important, and it is important for health care workers to use the hand hygiene methods appropriately. This aspect is critical to the project's success.

A very difficult aspect of this review is that only 2 studies qualified for inclusion, and the authors describe both as poorly controlled and inconclusive (Gould et al. 2007). A particular problem with the studies in this review was that follow-up was often limited to short periods of time, usually less than 6 months. While the recommendations for structuring research may be useful as the nurses evaluate the hand hygiene protocol, no recommendations for increasing adherence to such protocols were supported by research.

Level 3: Single Experimentally Designed Research Studies

There is a dearth of prospective clinical trials that evaluate the efficacy of hand hygiene practices and products. This area needs considerable work. The best controlled studies tend to be those assessing the effectiveness of alcohol rubs against antibiotic-resistant microbes. Rochon-Edouard et al. (2004) conducted a small comparative study testing four types of plated bacteria by exposing them to 9 different alcohol rub preparations. Additionally, 10 health care workers had their thumbprints sampled, followed by an alcohol rub, then re-sampled immediately after the rub and sampled again 5 minutes later. One alcohol rub was highly effective against the 4 bacteria and was also acceptable to the health care workers. The study was evidence Level 3, but the quality of evidence is at best medium. While the testing of the plated bacteria with alcohol gels was well controlled, the sample size of just 10 health care workers is quite small and may not have been representative of the greater population of health care workers.

Level 4: Systematic Reviews of Non-Experimental Studies

Once again, systematic reviews of non-experimental studies on hand hygiene protocols and practices are limited, although a portion of the systematic review that formed the basis for the CDC recommendation (Boyce and Pittet 2002) was composed of non-experimental studies.

Level 5: Single Non-Experimental or Qualitative Research Studies

A number of retrospective studies or descriptive studies regarding hand hygiene and hygiene products have been conducted. While each of these studies has limitations affecting their application, they nonetheless provide insight into the topic of hand hygiene. Box 10-4 shows a worksheet to assess an individual research study that was formatted as a retrospective chart review. The researchers examined alcohol gel use and nosocomial infection rates for orthopedic patients.

Other individual studies examined product assessment in terms of microbial activity as well as health care worker assessment of the products. Gordin, Schultz, Huber, and Gill (2005) conducted a 6-year observational survey at a tertiary, inner city medical center to assess the impact of using alcohol-based rubs in a clinical setting. The first 3 years of observation reflected no use while the final 3 years followed the introduction of alcohol-based gels. After implementation of the alcohol gel protocol, there was a 21% reduction in nosocomial methicillin resistant *Staphylococcus aureas* (MRSA) and a 41% decrease in vancomycin resistant *Enterococcus* (VRE). This study presents moderate evidence that alcohol gels can reduce infection rates for antibiotic resistant organisms.

In an observational before-and-after study, Winston, Felt, Huang, and Chambers (2004) found a reduction in ventilator-associated pneumonia (VAP) following the introduction of alcohol hand gel in the surgical intensive care unit. VAP decreased from 28.1 cases per 1,000 ventilator patient days to 13.2 cases per 1,000 ventilator patient days. While this is a Level 5 study, its evidence is persuasive that alcohol gels can decrease infection.

Hand hygiene techniques affect infection outcomes. Widmer and Dangel (2004) conducted a prospective study of 60 infection control specialists evaluating technique on the effectiveness of alcohol gel rubs. Fluorescent dye markers were added to hand antiseptics in order to identify missed areas following cleansing. Agar plates were used before and 1 minute after cleansing to assess bacterial counts. Following cleansing, one third of participants had no

BOX 10-4 Worksheet for Individual Research Study Appraisal

Citation:
Hilburn, J., B. Hammond, E. Fendler, and P. Groziak. 2003. Use of alcohol hand sanitizer as an infection control strategy in an acute care facility. *American Journal of Infection Control*, *31*(2): 109–116.

Summary:
List the purpose of the study (research questions, hypotheses, aims, or objectives).

- Examine infection rates and cost analysis before and after implementation of an alcohol gel rub hand hygiene protocol.

Identify the variables/phenomena.

- Infection: any nosocomial infection developed after 72 hours of admission including gastro-intestinal infections, respiratory infections, urinary tract infections, and bacteremias.

- Infection reduction: derived by subtracting average infection rate during the hand sanitizer period from the average rate of infection during the control period.

- Cost analysis

Identify the population and the sample.

- Population: Orthopedic surgical patients

- Sample: Orthopedic surgical patients at facility for 16-month period of study (6 months baseline and 10 months post introduction of alcohol gel protocol)

Identify the study design (experimental, non-experimental, or qualitative).

- Non-experimental, retrospective chart review

Describe any intervention or treatment.

- Protocol using alcohol gel rub instead of handwashing. Relatively extensive description of how protocol was carried out.

Identify sample number and sampling technique.

- Total sample number not specified; key component of calculations were based on patient days. Sampling technique: convenience; patients admitted to orthopedic unit.

Identify the instruments used.

- Infection identification via chart review.

Identify data analysis procedures (statistics or theme derivation process).

- Infection rates were calculated using number of infections during month divided by number of resident days in the month x 1,000.

- Cost analysis was conducted for costs associated with urinary tract infections (UTI). Financial records were reviewed for costs associated with UTI for both control and post treatment patients. Cost to charge ratio was determined by multiplying actual patient charges by 0.7 to estimate facility cost.

Describe the sample characteristics.

- Not described.

continued . . .

continued . . .
Summarize the results.

• Following the introduction of alcohol gel rubs, significant reductions occurred in all nosocomial infections with UTIs experiencing the greatest reduction. Infection rates were reduced from 8.2% to 5.3%, reducing the number of infections by 36% during the intervention period. Average savings were estimated at $91,257.57.

	Yes	No
Credibility:		
Was article peer reviewed?	X	
Was research problem clearly identified? Never directly stated, but implied through discussion of problem and methodology.		X
Were the research questions answered? Implied questions answered.	X	
Were the instruments reliable and valid? Standard methods for calculation used for infection rate and cost analysis.	X	
Was the sample large enough to find a significant outcome? Data represented a 16-month data collection; however, specific *n*'s were not reported—so it is difficult to assess sample size adequacy.		X
If statistics were used, were the findings significant? An ANOVA examining month by month infection rates before and after intervention was reported. ANOVA findings were not reported in article.	X	
Were the limitations of the study identified?		X
Applicability:		
Does the study examine your intervention or comparison intervention of interest? Probably the most directly related study in terms of problem of interest, population, and intervention.	X	
Does the study use a sample similar to your population of interest? The same type of population.	X	
Do the results help support your intervention of interest? Findings support the use of alcohol gel for nosocomial infection reduction.	X	

Evidence Level: Level 5   **Evidence Quality:** Medium

detectable bacteria on their skin. However, participants consistently missed some areas during antisepsis, particularly portions of the thumb and forefinger. Investigators concluded that technique matters when utilizing alcohol hand gels. A major difference in this study and the nurses' proposed intervention is that the study participants are infection control specialists rather than unit health care workers, who would be implementing the proposed protocol change.

Several studies regarding compliance with hand hygiene protocols have been conducted. Researchers usually measure adherence to protocols by observation or by measurement of the consumption of hand hygiene materials such as alcohol gels or antiseptic products. Herud, Nilsen, Svendheim, and Harthug (2009) utilized data from purchasing and admissions to assess the association between use of hand hygiene products and infection rates. As usage of hand hygiene products increased, infection rates decreased from 8% to 6%, a marginally significant finding. Investigators concluded that product utilization may serve as an indicator of hand hygiene performance in hospitals.

Howard et al. (2009) investigated if the introduction of a clean practice protocol (CPP) that incorporated hand hygiene and well as other practices would improve adherence to protocols. An audit system was developed to assess observed performance. An initial audit of the use of CPP was taken. Information from the audit was shared with the staff, followed by an education and awareness program that included signs posted at meetings and in common areas. Three months later a repeat audit was performed. Following the education and awareness program, hand hygiene significantly improved from the baseline of 28% to 87% across the surgical specialties. Investigators concluded that the education regarding CPPs was an effective method to improve practice. While this study provides some useful insight regarding education practices, the study lacked controls or a focus on clean practice behaviors beyond the 3-month follow-up period.

In an observational study, Wendt, Knautz, and von Braun (2004) examined how often health care workers followed their institution's protocol for using antiseptic hand rubs. Using the Fulkerson scale that rated fifteen health care activities, observers completed 2,138 observations of nurses and physicians working on general units or in the intensive care unit (ICU). Overall, hand rubs were used in 52% (1,115) of the total observations. Nurses used hand rubs significantly more often than physicians, and health care workers on general units used hand rubs more frequently than ICU workers. A major limitation of this study related to the intermittent nature of observations by forty-one different observers. While a standardized scale was used for behavior audit, there was no evidence presented regarding the reliability or validity of the instrument. Evidence level is low since there were no controls to study, although the concept of observation for adherence is potentially useful.

Braun, Kusek, and Larson (2009) conducted a field survey that tackled the issue of accurately measuring adherence to hand hygiene guidelines. Using a prepared list of essential hand hygiene attributes, the expert panel rated practices sent by 242 respondents who answered the call for effective measurement practices. Of the forty responses that met the screening criteria, only 12 were rated as good overall and 7 rated as promising. While a universal method of assessment was not found, authors made the following recommendations: (a) consider goals of measuring adherence, (b) use more than one approach for measurement, and (c) assess a variety of areas regarding hand hygiene such as staff knowledge, staff attitudes, and patient satisfaction. The nurses found information from this survey potentially useful in selecting methods to evaluate the new hand hygiene protocol.

Level 6: Non-Research Driven Expert Opinion or Committee Reports

Two non-research articles provided relevant information on the topic of hand hygiene. While these articles represent Level 6 information, the lowest level in the evidence hierarchy, they nonetheless provide some useful considerations for implementing a hand hygiene protocol. Bjerke (2004) traced the evolution of handwashing to hand hygiene by examining its importance with regard to infection control and prevention, facilities for handwashing, agents used for hand hygiene, product selection, indications for handwashing, preparation and methods of hand hygiene, and compliance. She concluded that when moving to alcohol rub use, (a) hand hygiene is an important care component for infection prevention, (b) hand hygiene needs to be valued by health care workers, and (c) facility-monitored personnel performance was critical to ensure effective hand hygiene programs.

Bush et al. (2007) offered a practical guide for installing hand hygiene products in a large health care system. Based on their experience, the authors recommend identifying and involving stakeholders, examining issues that affect product choice, planning ahead to address adverse reactions, planning for system maintenance, and communication. Although this article is Level 6 from an evidence perspective, it does contains key pieces of information that could prove useful in system implementation.

Consider This ...

How would you rate the evidence uncovered thus far? What steps would you recommend the nurses take next?

Step 4: Integrate the Evidence and Implement the Intervention

Now that the nurses have reviewed the individual pieces of evidence, it is time for them to put the whole picture together. Box 10-5 shows a worksheet for a Body of Evidence Appraisal, which summarizes the individual pieces of evidence available about hand hygiene. Worksheets such as this can help in the process of **evidence integration**.

With the strong recommendations of the CDC Guidelines (Boyce and Pittet 2002), as well as evidence that alcohol gels are effective against antibiotic-resistant organisms, the nurses decided to move forward to develop an alcohol gel protocol. Unfortunately, some of the research produced relatively weak levels of evidence. However, this project is a relatively low-risk intervention that will not be exceptionally expensive to introduce. Plus, it has the added benefits of time savings for health care workers and potential reduction of nosocomial infections. While it will take personnel effort to plan and implement the protocol, the time and effort that would need to be expended is not unreasonable.

Consider This ...

Do you agree with the nurses' decision to adopt use of alcohol gels? What would you have done when faced with this evidence, and why?

Because the CDC guidelines represent the standard of the industry, the nurses incorporated key pieces of their recommendations into their project. Based on the recommendations of Bush et al. (2007), they assembled a taskforce of representatives from the groups affected by the change—health care workers, a unit educator, purchasing, facilities management, housekeeping, and occupational health—to design the protocol and to plan for implementation.

The purpose of the alcohol gel protocol was two-fold: first, to provide an efficient mechanism for hand hygiene that would be more time effective than traditional handwashing and second, to provide effective nosocomial infection control for the unit's joint replacement patients.

The recommendations of the CDC Guidelines (Boyce and Pittet 2002) were readily transferrable to Hope Hospital and key steps were easy to incorporate into the protocol. The first part of the protocol addresses when hand hygiene should occur.

- Visibly soiled hands will be washed with either non-microbial or microbial soap and water.
- When hands are not visibly soiled, an alcohol gel hand rub will be used to decontaminate hands:

BOX 10-5 Worksheet for Body of Evidence Appraisal

	Yes	No
Intervention:		
Is patient safety a factor in implementing the intervention?		X

Patients should reap benefits from better hand hygiene. However, research shows that some health care workers may experience some side effects such as dermatitis from the hand care products.

	Yes	No
Is patient satisfaction a factor?		X

Patient satisfaction is not a factor; however, health care worker satisfaction may be a significant factor in terms of adherence to the new hand hygiene protocol.

What costs are associated with implementing the intervention?

- Costs associated with alcohol gel dispenser and supplies of alcohol gel.
- Personnel costs for installation and maintenance of dispensers as well as education time for health care providers to learn about new protocol.

What personnel resources are needed to implement the intervention?

- Unit educator: to teach health care workers about the new protocol.
- All unit health care workers: time for protocol education and for routine implementation.
- Purchasing department: product ordering for gel dispensers and gel.
- Maintenance: to install and maintain gel dispensers.
- Housekeeping: to replace alcohol gel packets when they are depleted.
- Occupational health: to devise a protocol for health care worker dermatitis (Bush et al. 2007).

Quality of Evidence:

How many Level 1-3 studies support the intervention?

- One clinical practice guideline issued by the CDC.
- One systematic review (limited support).
- Only one experimental study (part of study was experimental) (low).

How many Level 4-5 studies support the intervention?

Eight studies related to infection transmission, technique, and adherence.

What was the overall quality of the evidence? (high, medium, low)

Medium: While the CDC guideline is the strongest source of evidence and certainly recognized as the definitive practice standard, and the microbial studies regarding effectiveness against pathogens indicate alcohol gel effectiveness, studies regarding implementation, infection reduction, and particularly long-term adherence are not strong. Thus, the overall evidence level is low. One particularly applicable study was Hilburn et al. (2003) who studied alcohol gel use and infection in orthopedic patients. This study is rated as medium for its applicability.

Transferability:

	Yes	No
Are the populations in a majority of studies similar with the population at your institution?	X	

continued . . .

continued . . .	Yes	No
Is your institution similar to the study settings?	X	

Hope Hospital is an acute care institution which is similar to the sites of many of the studies. Only one study specifically examined orthopedic surgery patients. Other studies included surgical patients and intensive care patients.

How many participants would be affected by the intervention?
All health care workers on the orthopedic unit and the patients they care for.

Feasibility:

	Yes	No
Is there institutional support for the intervention?	X	

The institution is looking for ways to increase efficiency in care provision.

	Yes	No
Do staff have the skills to implement the intervention?		X

Staff currently practices handwashing. Education would be needed to ensure all health care workers know the key elements of the new protocol and understand the importance of implementation.

	Yes	No
Does the intervention add to staff workload?		X

Intervention should actually reduce staff work load since using alcohol gel would reduce the amount of time spent handwashing when entering a patient room.

What are possible barriers and facilitators to implementing this intervention?

Barriers:
- Health care workers dislike protocol or experience dermatitis from alcohol gel.
- Accurate methods for measuring adherence are not clearly delineated.

Facilitators:
- Use of gel saves health care worker time.
- Alcohol gel dispensers convenient to use.

Adopt___X___Consider a pilot project_____ Do not adopt_____

- Before direct contact with patients.
- When donning sterile gloves to insert central vascular catheter, indwelling urinary catheters, peripheral vascular catheters, or other nonsurgical invasive devices.
- After contact with patient's intact skin (such as taking blood pressures).
- After contact with body fluids.
- When moving from contaminated body site to a clean site.
- After contact with medical equipment.
- After removing gloves.
- Wash hands with either non-microbial or microbial soap and water before eating and after using the restroom.

The protocol also adopted specific techniques for hand hygiene outlined by the CDC (Boyce and Pittet 2002). For example:

For hand decontamination with alcohol-based rub:

- Apply rub to the palm of one hand (amount of rub determined by manufacturer's recommendation for product used);

- rub hands together in order to cover all surfaces on hands and fingers;
- rub until the hands are dry.

For soap and water handwashing:

- wet hands first with water (avoid using hot water because repeated washing may lead to dermatitis);
- apply soap (amount of soap determined by manufacturer's recommendation for product used);
- vigorously rub hands together covering all surfaces for at least fifteen seconds;
- thoroughly rinse;
- dry with a disposable paper towel;
- use towel to turn off the faucet.

The nurses developed plans for project implementation using the guidance offered by Bush et al. (2007). Key pieces of the process included the following tasks, with responsible parties indicated:

- Health care workers will have representatives on the taskforce and be consulted about the feasibility and acceptability of the protocol, including trying out sample devices and products.
- Infection Control representative will ensure that the new protocol fits within the institution's guidelines. He/she will also work to supply current unit infection information and track future infection rates for the unit. Representative may also make specific recommendations when selecting the alcohol gel rub product based on the efficacy of the selected rub.
- Purchasing representative will investigate the cost of the gel dispensing devices and the initial and continuing costs for supplying alcohol gel. Purchasing will be responsible for ordering the necessary supplies.
- Maintenance representative will develop a plan for installation of the gel devices and replacing broken or defective units.
- Housekeeping will develop a plan for routinely resupplying the gel devices when gel packets are empty.
- Unit educator will develop a program to explain the new hand hygiene protocol and make plans to ensure full staff participation. Based on the work of Howard et al. (2009), the program will include an initial educational offering as well as mechanisms such as unit signs to remind staff of the hand hygiene protocol.
- The Occupational health nurse will be responsible for devising a plan for preventing or dealing with dermatitis that may be associated with alcohol gel use for a small number of nurses and may also make recommendations for specific products that have a lower rate of dermatologic side effects.

With the key players in place, implementation of the protocol moved forward.

Step 5: Evaluate the Outcomes

The final piece of the EBP process is planning for **outcome evaluation**. Outcome evaluation is the process of determining the effectiveness of the evidence-based intervention. In the initial problem formulation, the key piece of outcome information sought was the unit infection rate. At best, it can be anticipated that using the alcohol gel rub protocol would improve infection rates (Gordin et al. 2005; Hilburn et al. 2003; Rochon-Edouard et al. 2004; Winston et al. 2004). One key piece of evidence would be to compare infection rates before and after 6 North adopts the hand hygiene protocol. Infection rates should be tracked not only immediately following the protocol change, but also should continue to be tracked for the unit over the long term.

Secondary concerns for the unit may be ensuring adherence to the protocol as well as assessing the acceptability of the change for health care workers. The findings of the Cochrane Database review by Gould et al. (2007) point to some of the difficulties in planning effective evaluation of protocol implementation. While there are standardized mechanisms for calculating infection rates (similar to those used by Hilburn et al. 2003), it was hard for the nurses to find viable measures of measures of protocol adherence (Braun et al. 2009). The nurses' recommendations include using more than one measure to assess adherence such as observation and measurement of cleaning product use. One strategy for observation studies is to do an audit of hand hygiene behaviors exhibited (Howard, et al. 2009; Wendt et al. 2004).

A final evaluation consideration is a cost/benefit analysis of making the change. How much did it cost the unit to switch to an alcohol gel system? What benefits have been derived? Were there fewer nosocomial infections? Did it in fact take each nurse less time on entering a patient's room to use alcohol gel rubs versus soap-and-water washing? The nurses found one example of estimating the cost of care in Hilburn et al. (2003): investigators examined the costs of treating urinary tract infections (UTIs), including factors such as length of additional stay, supplies and equipment, microbiology studies in laboratory, other laboratory costs, diagnostic tests, medications, and intravenous supplies. The nurses determined that Hope Hospital's business department could help provide figures associated with patient charges.

Consider This . . .

Why is evaluation such a critical piece of the EBP process? If you were conducting this process, what strategies would you use to make sure the evaluation was completed?

Step 6: Disseminate the Outcomes

Many wonderful projects that make a difference in health care fade into obscurity simply because the individuals involved failed to communicate the outcomes to others. The nurses on 6 North successfully planned, implemented, and evaluated an evidence-based project for their unit. Since the intervention was not expensive, reduced infection rates, and took less nursing time, the outcomes needed to be shared. The nurses shared outcomes initially with the administrators who suggested updating the hospital handwashing policy and implementing a hospital-wide change. To communicate to other nurses, they developed a poster for Hope Hospital's Evidence-Based Practice day. Additionally, they worked with the nursing education department to develop education materials for implementing a new handwashing policy hospital wide. Now they are contemplating an article about their experiences for a clinical journal. They also are eagerly looking forward to their next evidence-based project.

This chapter has presented a short example of the EBP process. Sample materials demonstrate the process that you might encounter when you move into the world of EBP. These tools are transferrable to many different settings and can help guide you as you make evidence-based decisions.

SUMMARY

- The evidence-based practice model uses a systematic process to evaluate interventions for clinical problems. The six steps of the evidence-based practice model are to (1) identify the clinical problems to form the question, (2) collect the evidence by searching the literature, (3) appraise the evidence, (4) integrate the evidence and implement the intervention, (5) evaluate the outcomes, and (6) disseminate the outcomes. Using the PICO(T) approach provides a useful template for stating a **clinical problem**. *(Objective 1)*

- Literature reviews consist of a systematic process beginning with (a) defining and refining a topic using search tools such as Boolean operators, (b) selecting appropriate resources, (c) choosing appropriate databases, (d) defining the search parameters and running a search, (e) examining the search results, and (f) collecting the resources found in the search. *(Objective 2)*

- Once literature is collected, a systematic **evidence appraisal** process can help determine the quality of the evidence under consideration. Worksheets facilitate the process of ranking the evidence on a 6-level hierarchy. *(Objective 3)*

- Following evidence appraisal, individual pieces of evidence must be put together into a larger picture. Worksheets can facilitate the **evidence integration** process. Intervention implementation must be planned using the evidence found and by strategizing with key players to address the complexities of the plan. *(Objective 4)*

- After intervention implementation, the process is followed by **outcome evaluation**. The plan must address how to measure the effects of the intervention in terms of outcomes as well as cost effectiveness. *(Objective 5)*

- The process is completed by disseminating the outcomes. A dissemination plan might include local venues such as a unit or the hospital. Nurses may also consider avenues such as poster or podium presentations at conferences or even writing about the implementation and outcomes of the project for a newsletter or journal for publication. *(Objective 6)*

STUDENT ACTIVITIES

In this chapter, you have followed an imaginary group of nurses as they worked through the process of evidence-based practice. Here are a couple of exercises that will help you gain experience in applying the EBP model.

1. With a class group, explore the evidence for accurately taking blood pressure. Go though the steps of the process from problem identification. Remember to develop a plan for implementation and a mechanism for measuring the outcomes. Think about where to disseminate findings.

2. When you are in your clinical setting, explore the hospital policy and procedure manual.
   a. Look for procedures that were developed using an evidence-based process.
   b. When you are on the unit, notice if staff are following the specified procedures.
   c. Think of ways to measure the outcomes of following the hospital's procedures.

3. In a clinical journal, find an evidence-based article that reports on a clinical practice.

   a. Does the journal explain the process used to evaluate the practice?
   b. Did authors indicate how the evidence-based plan was implemented?
   c. How might you evaluate the usefulness of the practice?

Pearson Nursing Student Resources

Find additional review materials at

www.nursing.pearsonhighered.com

Prepare for success with additional NCLEX®-style practice questions, interactive assignments and activities, web links, animations and videos, and more!

REFERENCES

Bjerke, N. 2004. The evolution: Handwashing to hand hygiene guidance. *Critical Care Nursing Quarterly,* *27*(2): 295–307.

Boyce, J. and D. Pittet. 2002. Guideline for hand hygiene in health-care settings: Recommendations of the Healthcare Infection Control Practices Advisory Committee and the HICPAC/SHEA/APIC Hand Hygiene Task Force. *Morbidity and Mortality Weekly Report, 51*(No. RR-16): 1–45. http://www.cdc.gov/handhygiene/Guidelines.html

Braun, B., L. Kusek, and E. Larson. 2009. Measuring adherence to hand hygiene guidelines: A field survey for examples of effective practices. *American Journal of Infection Control, 37*(4): 282–288.

Bush, K., M. Mah, G. Meyers, P. Armstrong, J. Stoesz, and S. Strople. 2007. Going dotty: A practical guide for installing new hand hygiene products. *American Journal of Infection Control, 35*(10): 690–693.

Gordin, F., M. Schultz, R. Huber, and J. Gill. 2005. Reduction in nosocomial transmission of drug-resistant bacteria after introduction of an alcohol-based hand rub. *Infection Control and Hospital Epidemiology, 26*(7): 650–653.

Gould, D., J. Chudleigh, D. Moralejo, and N. Drey. 2007. Interventions to improve hand hygiene compliance in patient care. *Cochrane Database of Systematic Reviews,* Issue 2. Art. No.:10.1002/14651858.CD005186.pub2.

Herud, T., R. Nilsen, K. Svendheim, and S. Harthug. 2009. Association between use of hand hygiene products and rates of health care associated infections in a large university hospital in Norway. *American Journal of Infection Control, 37*(4): 311–317.

Hilburn, J., B. Hammond, E. Fendler, and P. Groziak. 2003. Use of alcohol hand sanitizer as an infection control strategy in an acute care facility. *American Journal of Infection Control, 31*(2): 109–116.

Howard, D., C. Williams, S. Sen, A. Shah, J. Baurka, R. Bird, A. Loh, and A. Howard. 2009. A simple effective clean practice protocol significantly improves hand decontamination and infection control measures in the acute surgical setting. *Infection, 37*(1): 34–38.

Larsen, E.L. 1995. APIC guideline for handwashing and hand antisepsis in health care settings. *American Journal of Infection Control, 23*(4): 251–269.

Melnyk, B. and E. Fineout-Overholt. 2011. *Evidence based practice in nursing and health care* (2nd ed.). New York, NY: Lippincott Williams & Wilkins.

Rochon-Edouard, S., J. Pons, B. Veber, M. Larkin, S. Vassal, and J. Lemeland. 2004. Comparative in vitro and in vivo study of nine alcohol-based hand rubs. *American Journal of Infection Control, 32*(4): 200–204.

Wendt, C., D. Knautz, and H. von Baum. 2004. Differences in hand hygiene behavior related to the contamination risk of healthcare activities in different groups of healthcare workers. *Infection Control and Hospital Epidemiology, 25*(3): 203–206.

Widmer, A. and M. Dangel. 2004. Alcohol based hand rub: Evaluation of technique and microbiological efficacy with international infection control professionals. *Infection Control and Hospital Epidemiology, 25*(3): 207–209.

Winston, L., S. Felt, W. Huang, and H. Chambers. 2004. Introduction of a waterless hand gel was associated with a reduced rate of ventilator associated pneumonia in a surgical intensive care unit. *Infection Control and Hospital Epidemiology, 25*(12): 1015–1016.

Index

Note: Page numbers followed by "*f*" indicate a figure; those followed by "*b*" indicate a box; and those followed by "*t*" indicate a table.